Endorsements

"Everyone needs to read this book! Ms. Michael's story is a guide to self-induced healing that can help anyone be prepared and not have to learn from personal disaster. Cancer can be a wake-up call to a new beginning as it was for Ms. Michaels. In her powerful story of rebirth, we learn that amazing things can happen when our body gets the message that we are living a new life we love."

> Dr. Bernie Siegel, MD, author of *The Art of Healing* and *A Book of Miracles*

"*The Gift of Cancer* is an inspiring and deep personal history of how cancer closed some doors but opened so many others, leading to personal transformation and growth. The strength and empowerment of taking control of your health and treatment plan, staying committed, and coming out the other side stronger and healthier will inspire many in similar situations. I highly recommended this book to anyone struggling with any major life issue."

> Joel Kahn MD, Professor of Medicine, Wayne State University School of Medicine, Director Cardiac Wellness, Michigan Healthcare Professionals, PC

"This book is a roadmap for anyone challenged with dis-ease. Facing incredible odds, Brenda Michaels made the courageous decision to embrace her cancer as her "teacher" rather than as her enemy. In doing so, she was guided to heal her inner life, which led to the healing of her cancer."

> Marci Shimoff, professional speaker, bestselling author, *Happy for No Reason, Love For No Reason, Chicken Soup for the Woman's Soul*

"Brenda Michaels, with Marsha Mercant tells her story with such openness and courage. It will resonate with anyone who is struggling to trust her inner voice. I couldn't put it down! I will keep this book by my bed—to remind me that I am the only one who can heal myself."

Jill Eikenberry, actor, breast cancer activist

"Brenda Michaels' story is one that will resonate with every human being. In her book, *The Gift of Cancer: A Miraculous Journey to Healing*, Ms. Michaels shares how her experience with cancer propelled her to look deep within her heart to access love, faith and ultimately forgiveness. We all struggle with judgment and fear, not realizing how that can impact our health, relationships and the very fabric of our lives. This book is a beautifully written story of hope and inspiration; a testimonial to the power of love within each of us."

Dr. DiVanna VaDree DC, CA, CIH, Full Body Channel for Divine Mother Quan Yin

"Brenda Michaels' story is an inspiration to us all. It is a story of success against terrible odds, of quiet moments of courage and heroism in times of fear and doubt. I recommend this book to everyone, to those whose life is difficult for any reason, for those facing a cancer diagnosis, for anyone who wants an uplifting story of a woman's courage and triumph over some very serious battles. I admire Brenda for sharing this very personal story and for the successful life she has created for herself. "

Nicholas J. Gonzalez, M.D.

"This book is a miracle, providing an example of someone claiming her true spiritual power in the midst of challenges and healing into who she is meant to be. *The Gift of Cancer* is a tender, passionate, instructive tale that is a gift to anyone."

Tama Kieves, bestselling author of *Inspired & Unstoppable: Wildly Succeeding in Your Life's Work!* www.TamaKieves.com

"Brenda Michaels' book, *The Gift of Cancer*, is a gift of deep wisdom and compassion to all who suffer, be it from physical illness, emotional pain or spiritual bewilderment. Her profound journey into the heart of serious illness is a testament to her raw courage and faith in the greater mystery of life's unfolding. Through Brenda's robust description of her extraordinary experience, we discover new and surprising possibilities for our own healing and wholeness; truths that offer us a larger, life-changing perspective of our most essential selves."

Susan Plummer, Ph.D, author of *Deep Change: Befriending the Unknown*

"*The Gift of Cancer* by Brenda Michaels with Marsha Mercant is a gem of a book! If you are at a health crossroads, seeking a new perspective that offers hope and possibility using an alternative path to healing of the mind, body, spirit, this book is especially for you. If you or a loved one are looking for insight as you explore the physical, emotional and spiritual implications of wellness and are desiring new tools and support to move through turbulent times, this book is well worth the read and highly recommended.

Robin Mastro, author of *Altars of Power and Grace, Making Room for Mr. Right*, environmental designer, teacher of Vedic Knowledge

"This book needs to be read; by women fighting breast cancer, by anybody, man or woman dealing with any type of cancer, by anyone seeking a wonderfully written, passionately told story of an unusual woman coming to age and into good health – a woman who followed her own good instincts along the way and sought out expert guides to help in her quest."

Suzanne Somers, actor, health activist

"Brenda Michaels, with Marsha Mercant has written a beautiful, painful work of heart. She teaches us how to heal, making the physical aspects of disease disappear in the harmony of wholeness and self-realization. Brenda's determination is awe inspiring as she cultivates peace within pain, harmony through faith and the courage to follow intuitive wisdom regardless of outside opinion. This profound journey will remind every reader what they are capable of!"

Holly Riley, inspirational speaker, bestselling author of *Allowing: A Portrait of Forgiving and Letting Life Love You*

"This book is a must read for anyone faced with the life changing journey of cancer. Through her personal story, Brenda Michaels brings a unique blend of hope and understanding to the conversation of terminal illness, exploring an array of possibilities that can be found just outside the paradigm of traditional medicine."

Royce Richardson, author of *The Blissmaker*

"Brenda Michaels with Marsha Mercant, has written a beautiful book for anyone reflecting on her own spiritual path. For those challenged with illness, there is important information about creating a healing team, managing fears and moving positively into the light of health and happiness. By embracing cancer as a teacher instead of the enemy Brenda offers an amazing lesson to us all. I gleaned so many pearls of wisdom that I have put in my journal so I may reflect on them when I forget to trust the divine. "

Mary Ann Halpin, photographer, creator of *Fearless Women, Visions of a New World*, *Pregnant Goddesshood* and Fearless Women series

"Reading Brenda Michaels' story was life changing for me. I've never had cancer but I do have relationships that have been emotionally painful and toxic. After reading this book, I've begun a daily regimen of morning meditation to re-examine, release and re-center. What an amazing gift this book is!"

Sharon Carr, Tony Award–winning Broadway producer

"Brenda Michaels' *The Gift of Cancer: A Miraculous Journey to Healing* is a story of not only healing but ultimately, empowerment. As we witness Ms. Michaels not only survive but thrive through three cancer diagnoses, she is an inspiration and testament to the power of facing your fears. Her story is real and honest as she encounters fear, grief, failure, shame and loss moving from victim to creator. In the face of great obstacles we witness her reclaim her life, find her voice and heal her soul, achieving the peace and joy she longs for."

Megan Skinner, spiritual counselor and author

"Congratulations on *The Gift of Cancer: A Miraculous Journey to Healing*. I think you have a hit on your hands! And not just because it's something everyone will want to read, but because it's something everyone SHOULD read! You can quote me on that!"

David Friedman, award-winning composer, author of *Thought Exchange*

"This story of courage and healing demonstrates the power of the author's remarkable commitment to accept and receive the lessons of her cancer diagnosis. As she learned to surrender, to trust, and to practice forgiveness, soul-level healing was made possible. For those who are ready to hear her message, the inspiration she offers can open doorways to life-affirming possibilities and activate unrealized healing potential."

Madeline Eyer, author of *Essential Green Smoothies*

"*The Gift of Cancer* spoke deeply to me, as a woman and artist. It was reminiscent of how I felt after reading *Eat, Pray, Love*, which plugged me into myself in profound ways. But the journey Brenda Michaels takes to heal her cancer and rid herself of negative responses to the ups and downs of life, speaks to an audience that is yearning for a deeper connection and ultimate healing. It is an amazing story of triumph. I would love to see it as a film, a television series or even a hosted talk show!"

Sumer Crockett Moore, award-winning actor, producer

"*The Gift of Cancer: A Miraculous Journey to Healing* takes the reader on a remarkable and inspiring journey through cancer and Brenda Michaels' own awakening to the healing powers of body, mind and spirit. A must read for anyone desiring to live her highest and best life."

DS Clark, author of *The Stone Ones* trilogy

"This illuminating book speaks to the profound choice between taking responsibility or being a victim. It shows us the empowering nature of taking personal responsibility for one's life and by that act our path is enlightened."

Dr. Robert Abramson, MD, Master of Acupuncture

"*The Gift of Cancer* takes us on a very personal healing journey of self-discovery with unexpected twists and insights along the way. We witness dysfunctional relationships that set the stage for the development of multiple cancers to equally pathological interactions with the conventional medical system. After many frustrating setbacks, magical synchronicities eventually provide guidance into the realms of nutritional cancer therapy and spiritual transformation. This insightful book offers valuable lessons about surrender and self-healing for all of us."

Larry Burk, MD, CEHP, author of *Let Magic Happen: Adventures in Healing with a Holistic Radiologist*

"When I was a young internal medicine doctor, a patient would occasionally say to me, 'Cancer is the best thing that ever happened to me.' Not understanding, I thought, *People will go to any length to put a good face on a terrible situation.* I eventually learned what my patients were telling me. We are more than a collection of organs; we are more than molecules; we are a whole and we are holy—words that are related to health and healing. And sometimes it takes a health crisis to awaken us to these truths.

"Brenda Michaels has lived this path. The spiritual, psychological, and physical integration she achieved is a talisman for the healing journey. *The Gift of Cancer* will inspire anyone who is fortunate enough to read it. But don't wait until you have a health crisis, because this wisdom is for everyone."

Larry Dossey, MD, author of *One Mind: How Our Individual Mind Is Part of a Greater Consciousness and Why It Matters*

THE GIFT OF CANCER

THE GIFT OF CANCER

A MIRACULOUS JOURNEY TO HEALING

BRENDA MICHAELS

WITH

MARSHA MERCANT

Foreword by Dr. Christiane Northrup

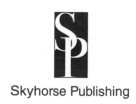

Skyhorse Publishing

Skyhorse Publishing books may be purchased in bulk at special discounts for sales promotion, corporate gifts, fund-raising, or educational purposes. Special editions can also be created to specifications. For details, contact the Special Sales Department, Skyhorse Publishing, 307 West 36th Street, 11th Floor, New York, NY 10018 or info@skyhorsepublishing.com.

Skyhorse® and Skyhorse Publishing® are registered trademarks of Skyhorse Publishing, Inc.®, a Delaware corporation.

Visit our website at www.skyhorsepublishing.com.

10 9 8 7 6 5 4 3 2

Library of Congress Cataloging-in-Publication Data is available on file.

Cover design by Eve Siegel
Cover photo credit Thinkstock

Print ISBN: 978-1-62914-571-6
Ebook ISBN: 978-1-62914-964-6

Printed in the United States of America

Acknowledgments

Brenda Michaels

I didn't consciously set out to write my story. And while birthing this book has been both exhilarating and laborious, I can now clearly see how the encouragement of friends pointed me to this destiny. Their support helped me understand that the book's message could potentially help those who struggle with chronic issues in their lives, particularly illness.

The catalyst I needed to write the first draft was Vishara Veda. Without her initial phone call and insistence, putting me together with my husband, this book would not exist. Thank you, Vishara, for your vision and your friendship.

To my amazing life partner and husband, Rob Spears. Your patience, insights, and writing skills moved this project forward. I am and will forever be grateful for everything you are and everything you bring to my life.

I want to also thank Phillip DeFranco, Royce Richardson, and Andrea Hurst. All three talented writers who in the early stages helped me put my book in order. Many times when my frustration was so great, thinking it would never be published, they helped me change my perspective so I could carry on. Your support and friendship mean the world to me.

To all my beloved friends: DiVanna VaDree, Megan Skinner, Maddy Eyer, Diana Clark, Dr. Shima Silber, Robin Mastro, and Karen Porter—your friendship and support through all the ups and downs of my journey have been incredible. You are truly my Soul Sisters. I am forever grateful for your presence in my life.

Last but by no means least, to two remarkable women who in a very short time have touched my life deeply—my wonderful agent, Lisa Hagan, and my amazing co-writer, Marsha Mercant. The moment I met each of these ladies there was an instant connection, and I recognized that they too were my Soul Sisters. Working with them is a gift I will forever cherish.

Acknowledgments

Marsha Mercant

First and foremost, I am forever grateful to Brenda Michaels for trusting me with her story. In retrospect, I can see that fate brought us together to create this book. It has been an honor and a delight to work with her and help bring her miraculous story to the world.

I must also thank Mary Ann Halpin who helped get me started on this most unexpected journey to becoming a writer. I could not have known when I agreed to co-edit one of her books, the treasures that would come out of that experience.

Also, to my husband, John Howard Swain, who believes in me even when I sometimes doubt myself. Who always has my best interests foremost in his thoughts. And who holds my heart with tender loving care that I may go out into the world and discover the things that sing to my soul.

To Marianna Dworak, who shepherded our manuscript with care and vision. To Lisa Hagan, our literary agent and friend, who has been our greatest cheerleader from day one and has lovingly answered every ridiculous question I've thrown her way.

And lastly, to Spirit, the great force that moves in mysterious ways, reminding me how much bigger His dreams for me are and encouraging me to move in the direction of my heart.

Dedications

Brenda Michaels:

First and foremost, I dedicate this book to Divine Mother, my guiding light, mentor, and loving presence that is always with me. Without her constant love, my life would be empty.

Secondly, I dedicate this work to two people who have loved and supported me on this journey—my beloved husband, friend, and life partner Rob, who has never wavered in his support of my growth and this project. I treasure his faith in me as well as his vision for us in service to a greater good.

And to my dear mother, who from the beginning has been one of my greatest cheerleaders. I deeply appreciate her willingness to listen to my truth, trusting that love and forgiveness heals all.

Marsha Mercant:

For Melinda Moreno Miller, my angel in life and ever after. Your grace, love, and courage opened my heart to unimagined possibility. Until we meet again . . .

Foreword

Written by Christiane Northrup, MD, bestselling author of *Women's Bodies, Women's Wisdom*, and *The Wisdom of Menopause*

We live in a culture in which most women's number one health concern and fear is breast cancer. Almost no one has the courage to look this disease in the eye and call it a gift. Almost no one, that is, except a few brave and compassionate souls like Brenda Michaels, who know from the inside out the secret of true healing because they've been there.

Brenda is a stunningly beautiful woman I met in San Diego several years ago. She had the courage to come up on stage during my presentation and tell her story of cancer recovery to the whole audience. Though Brenda followed a healthy diet and also had some conventional medical treatments, she knew full well that it wasn't simply a diet or a drug that had healed her various cancers. It was something else—her own inner wisdom and the consistent application of its messages in her life.

Brenda's story holds the key to approaching breast cancer, cervical cancer, or any other disease for that matter, with maximum access to our inner healing power. The first step we must all take in order to put this power to work in our lives is to tell the truth to ourselves about our lives without whitewashing it, cleaning it up to make it more acceptable, or wallowing in self-blame. Brenda does this admirably throughout *The Gift of Cancer*. In the beginning, when she was first diagnosed with cancer, she wrote, "Our marriage was filled with painful experiences reinforcing my belief that love hurts. To compensate, I gradually became a martyr, overextending myself constantly trying to please him, while disregarding my own needs and desires. True to form, I continued to manifest physical problems."

I've never met a single person, including myself, who has not faced challenges in the areas of personal relationships and physical health, two areas that are intimately related. Yet the vast majority of people are in denial about the implications of these life challenges, and when it comes to their health, put far too much faith in modern medicine while avoiding the core beliefs and behaviors that are at the root of their problems in the first place.

But every so often, one person, like Brenda Michaels, will find within herself the courage to really look at her life, embrace it, warts and all, and then change her beliefs and behaviors. And when this happens, she heals at the deepest levels. And many times, such as in Brenda's case, her body will heal as well. The end result is the greatest gift that anyone can give to the planet: a healed life. Brenda Michaels has healed her life. Let the wisdom she has gleaned spill over into your own life, so that you too can become healthy and whole.

TABLE OF CONTENTS

Introduction

The Gift

At age twenty-six I was given an unusual gift: cancer. I don't say this to make light of what appeared to be an early death sentence. Cancer devastated my life. My marriage was ripped apart and our meager finances were drained away faster than we could have imagined. Over the course of fourteen years, cancer claimed my entire reproductive system, both my breasts, and left me with a prognosis of one year to live. That was twenty-four years ago.

While cancer ushered in one of the most difficult periods of my life, it also ignited one of the most profound. Having cancer left me stranded in a place where no doctor had the capacity to save me. But it led me to the truth of who I am and the realization that only I possessed the power to save myself.

Forced to examine my life in new and challenging ways by the dramatic changes generated by my cancer diagnoses, I came to the understanding that if you are inclined to look for the silver lining amongst the dark clouds, you will find it. I learned that in the storm of crisis that is the healing process, there is enormous opportunity for growth and change. Those dark clouds of adversity have the power to strengthen, bring clarity, and reveal to us the miracles that lie beyond our limited beliefs. I now appreciate the importance of embracing that adversity as the gift it is. I finally know that those challenging experiences are a crucial piece of the puzzle that can serve our growth and transformation. Arriving at that knowing was not easy.

Life will consistently bring to light what is needed to nudge us toward the growth necessary for our highest good. And in perfect harmony with each life plan, every experience comes forth at the perfect moment to teach us something profound about ourselves. When we accept our challenges and move through the lessons inherent in them, we discover that healing energy is available to us, offering the hope of wholeness and an amazing future alive with possibility.

For me, the first step was to surrender to those lessons being called forth by my own being. To embrace what was in front of me so it could be transformed, thus fulfilling my deepest desire—for my life to be different.

As I moved toward that goal, a stark realization came into view. I had been living my life as a victim rather than a creator. And to be a victim, there must be a perceived persecutor. In my case, I believed my persecutors to be family, friends, and a husband cut from the same cloth as my father. With my belief in victimhood firmly in place, I felt powerless. Yet as much as I wanted to change this feeling, I couldn't seem to step out of my victim role. That is until cancer entered my life for the third time and opened my eyes to a universal truth: I am responsible for my life circumstances and my reactions to those circumstances. To continue to turn away or hide from the stressful signals I had been getting for years was no longer an option.

This was a hard pill to swallow. Especially when taking responsibility included not only for my circumstances, but also for my decisions and even my illness. There are those who will argue they are genetically predisposed to disease and are therefore victims of their illness. Logically and emotionally, this can be justified. I certainly don't debate that. I do, however, believe it is our inability to face stressful situations that fuel our problems and remove the possibility of transformation and healing.

When we ignore the signals that stressful events present, or believe we are helpless to change our circumstances, or fail to take responsibility for stress that is in our lives, we become victims to that situation. Once this happens, our ego-mind takes over and promises us solutions. But the ego-mind is not equipped to find solutions. Solutions can only be accessed through creative energy and an awareness of ourselves as spiritual beings.

The ego-mind loves to spin negative stories that offer countless band-aid solutions in support of our powerless victim mentality. Living in this limited capacity creates enormous stress on our bodies, which in turn triggers biological responses that can weaken our immune system's ability to access its healing energy. Living this way takes us down the path of heartache, disappointment, and inevitably, illness.

It is a medically documented fact that prolonged, unaddressed stress can lead to chronic illness. If we don't acknowledge this stress and ask what is needed of us in any given situation to alleviate it, we remain cut off from the wisdom of our hearts where all creative solutions are found.

When we are in reaction mode rather than response mode, we tend to do one of three things that exacerbate our situation: we either internalize the stress denying we are responsible for the circumstance; we avoid the situation altogether; or we numb ourselves so we don't have to deal with our feelings. The key to solving this is to face the problem, embrace it, and surrender to the strong emotions the problem triggers. By doing this, we create a space for our creative spirit to offer long-term solutions that lead to healing.

Once I realized I was running from my problems, I began to question if this might be one of the reasons I had fallen into the abyss of cancer. Asking this question pushed me to look at myself honestly. What I saw was someone who felt powerless to change the stressful events passing through her life. During stressful times, I would either internalize my feelings, denying what was going on, or I would numb myself with alcohol and drugs to quell the fear and pain coursing through me.

Once this process was in motion, judgment about my inability to deal with my situation would kick in and feelings of shame, guilt, and anger would flood my system. Then I would systematically punish myself for being weak by sabotaging everything good that came into my life.

Does this pattern sound familiar? How often do we punish ourselves for not knowing better, for not making a smarter decision? How often do we heap guilt and shame on ourselves, destroying our lives because we feel powerless and ashamed? How often do we turn away from our problems instead of engaging in potential solutions?

Once the awareness of these patterns took hold in me, I became passionate about finding out what drove them. I began to ask myself questions: What do I believe? How do I perceive the circumstances of my life? What are my dominant thought patterns? What began to emerge was a picture of a child that, like most children, took on her parents' beliefs, perceptions, fears, and doubts. This is what we do as children. We develop attitudes, beliefs, ways of dealing with problems and challenges based on the beliefs, perspectives and coping mechanisms we observe in our parents. Then we carry these observed "skills" into adulthood.

Most people are unaware of the profundity of this process because the patterns we develop sit in our unconscious. It is imperative, if we are to have any hope of changing our lives for the better, that we become aware of the negative beliefs, fears, and perspectives we take on as children. When we awaken to these patterns, we can begin to transform them, thus creating the opportunity to live our lives as empowered beings rather than victims.

For me, it took being diagnosed with my third bout of cancer before I was willing to look beyond the physical reasons for my disease and discover the deeper beliefs, perceptions, and emotional issues at the core of my illness. Over time, these issues, left unattended, created fertile ground for cancer to thrive in my body. It took the stark realization that I could die in a year's time for me to face the unacknowledged stresses contributing to my disease.

One of the first steps in healing anything in our lives is to *accept right where we are*. This is especially true if where we are is not where we want to be. We cannot heal what we deny or are unwilling to accept. By denying what begs our attention, we create resistance. We then give power to that resistance and, as we all know, what we resist persists!

For years, I resisted taking responsibility for my problems, my health, or my inability to stand in my own truth. Following the patterns established by my parents, I was afraid to confront the anger and fear that coursed through me. I had learned that problems are caused by something or someone outside myself. I used blame and criticism to point the finger in another direction. Others needed to change, not me.

To distract myself from taking responsibility for my actions, I kept busy. When that didn't work, I drank, watched too much television, or ate too much sugar. That did work, for a while. But "fixes" that originate in the ego-mind cannot last. What I perceived as coping strategies only led to my feeling powerless. It began to dawn on me that I must stop denying my feelings and blaming others. It was time to start looking inside myself for the answers to my problems.

Making this important decision created an environment where growth could take place—an atmosphere where I could transform my experiences into gifts of peace, healing, and wellbeing. As my commitment to this work took hold, a part of me began to awaken, what I call a *spiritual awakening*. But make no mistake, it takes work, hard work, and a deep desire to heal your life as much as you desire to heal your cancer, or whatever illness your body may be expressing.

The fear we carry about most disease is born in our lack of understanding of the power we possess to transform our lives. This knowledge is obscured by our distorted belief that we are powerless human beings rather than powerful God beings with the ability to transform and change our circumstances. We push away our ability to love and be loved. We live fast-paced, stressed-out lives. We eat lousy diets. We live in an environment that has been poisoned. Yes, genetic makeup can be a factor, but it is not the deciding factor. We are the deciding factor.

When allowed the proper environment, the body will always gravitate towards health. It's not only my responsibility to expose my body to the environment in which it can thrive, it is also a gift I can give myself each and every day.

My story is not only about healing the cancer that threatened my life, but also about the transformation I experienced beyond my physical condition. Whether it was relationship issues or financial devastation, coming to terms with my reality became the gifts that transformed my world and ultimately my health.

In the beginning stages of my diagnosis, I fought the cancer invading my body with a vengeance. Like most people, I wanted only one thing: to be rid of it. But over time, I realized this approach was not working. The cancer did go into remission for long periods of time, only to recur more severely. The third time I was diagnosed and told I wouldn't survive much past a year without chemotherapy, I was devastated. But this time, instead of repeating the pattern of turning away from my problems and depending on doctors to cure me, the healer in me began to awaken. I needed to get real about what was happening in my life and set a course for wellness.

It was in the early stages of this third diagnosis that I made the decision to embrace my cancer and allow it to teach me what I needed to learn. I made a commitment to heal my body of this disease once and for all. My desire to not only get well, but to create a harmonious body, mind, spirit connection became my passion. Once that passion was ignited, an internal shift began to take place.

I learned there is a distinct difference between healing and curing. Healing denotes a movement toward harmony with the body, mind, and spirit. Curing, on the other hand, is a means to an end. Curing a disease implies the disease is gone. But it begs the question: gone forever, or gone temporarily?

Healing involves the exploration and transformation of core issues that lead to illness. This exploration is done to move the physical disease-causing factors out of the body, transforming the consciousness that allowed the manifestation of disease in the first place. We must heal the negative thoughts and beliefs that threaten to contaminate our bodies. We must change the diets that poison and weaken our immune system. And we must eliminate the chemical toxins and other ecological factors that destroy our environment and our bodies.

When I was first diagnosed with cancer, healing was not part of my consciousness. I wanted only one thing—to be cured. I was scared, confused, and angry at my body's betrayal. I searched for a doctor who would give me answers and not only *fix* me, but also take responsibility for making me well. But after a long, exhaustive search with no lasting results, it dawned on me that the surgical procedures and recommended drugs were methods meant to treat my symptoms only. They were not meant to stop the cancer for good. The *fixes* being offered were temporary at best, aimed at *curing* the cancer rather than *healing* the whole of me. These methods were not targeted at the underlying issues that helped create the imbalance and the opportunity for disease to appear in the first place. In this realization was born a deep foreboding that I was unable to shake—this model of treating disease would not be enough to stop the assault on my body.

I realized the choices and decisions I'd made throughout my life had led to this moment. Perhaps, I thought, my past experience might hold the key to my present circumstance. Maybe by looking more closely at my life history, I might be able to better understand the beliefs that had determined my choices. If I could understand the how and why of my decisions, why I believed certain things about myself and my world, why my system felt so overwhelmed all the time, it might give me a foundation from which to work. I knew diving into my past would not be a pleasant journey. Nevertheless, it was the journey I had to take if I was going to heal my cancer and reclaim my life. For me, it was now or never.

Part One

Living in the Dark

1

Journey to the Past

Looking honestly at my life to the point where healing my cancer became my passion, I realized pain and struggle had been central themes. Once confronted with an unpleasant problem or situation, I would go into fight or flight mode. For days on end I would ruminate about how life was unfair and no one understood me. So convinced that life was against me, I created more and more problems to support my theory.

Lacking any insight into what I was doing or why I processed things the way I did, I had no hope of transcending this pattern. After years of living this way, I was exhausted. I started to believe life wasn't worth living. Then, without warning, came my third diagnosis of cancer, and immediately the words "careful what you wish for" flashed through my mind.

Although I had been contemplating the idea of ending the struggle once and for all, when it came right down to it, I wanted to live. Now, I actually had to do something about it. I started to ask myself questions I had never asked before: Why do I struggle every day with the simplest of problems? Why am I afraid to face my life? Why can't I be happy? Why am I bent on destroying myself? Granted, these were tough questions, but in retrospect, I realize that because of my willingness to face my fears, I was beginning to open to the possibility that this journey might lead me to the heart of my disease.

I somehow knew the only way to uncover the answers to these questions was to look into my past. The first image that came to mind was me, at age seven. That's when I realized I was different from other people, especially my family. Two brothers—one older, one younger—and a controlling father didn't leave much room for a sensitive intuit.

I was the child who challenged my parents, seeing and feeling things that others in my family didn't even acknowledge. My life was a series of stifled emotions and unexpressed feelings that caused me to act out. My behavior was confusing and seemed irrational to my frustrated parents, leading them to dub me the "troublemaker." With this label continually affirmed, I began to believe it. I also believed the companion thought, that there must be something wrong with me. These concepts took hold, shaping my behavior, and I came to accept that I was a bad person.

A large part of my childhood was spent trying to protect myself from my angry, controlling, volatile father whose use of a belt was his way of communicating. At the same time, I tried to get my emotionally detached mother to respond to my needs. It wasn't until after my father's death that I learned my mother was as lonely and scared as I was. This was the main reason she wasn't emotionally available when I needed her. She couldn't be there for herself, let alone for me. My father's passing gave us the opportunity to discuss many issues between us that had been dismissed. Thankfully, this brought with it the healing I craved, and now we have a healthy, loving relationship rooted in emotional honesty and compassion.

But I had grown up with fear as a constant predator in our house—fear of not having enough, fear of not being good enough, of failing, of never doing anything right, of losing our home. I came to learn it was these un-confronted fears that motivated all the decisions my parents made. We were taught that life was hard and struggle was a given.

It wasn't until I entered high school that I discovered my father had grown up in a poor family with an alcoholic, abusive father and a mother who was withdrawn and angry. Although my father rarely spoke about his childhood, whenever he did, it was painfully obvious he was ashamed of his upbringing and what he had become. While this was no excuse for his fits of anger and violent behavior, knowing this about him helped me understand why he was enraged with the world. It also helped me forgive him before he died.

My mother also came from a poor and abusive family. However, her abuse was more emotional than physical. Her father ruled his family very much like my father ruled ours. When Mom was young, she was taught that a woman's place was behind her husband, and if she questioned that position, she would be exposed to various forms of punishment. Thus, she took on the belief that women are second-class citizens to be seen and not heard. No surprise that this is what she taught me as well.

Due to my father's demanding nature and need to control everything, he had a tremendous impact on me as a child. Watching him struggle with the circumstances and events in his life continually affirmed for me that life demanded more than anyone was capable of giving. He reinforced that people are basically powerless to change their circumstances. He also taught me that he was always right.

And although there were a number of good things he taught me, especially when it came to extending kindness to others, it was the things that made me feel small, afraid, and powerless that imprinted deeply on my psyche. My mother is also very kind and did her best to protect us from my father when he would rant. But she had learned it was imperative to please others, and in the end would give in to him.

As I witnessed my mother's constant sacrifice, I learned to disregard my own needs and wants for the needs and wants of others. Once out on my own, this pattern continued with all my relationships, resulting in my resentment of the very people I tried so hard to please. What I didn't realize at the time was my so-called sacrifice was really for my own selfish gain. I did things for others to get two things for me: their love and devotion. The irony is that I never felt that I received those, which only served to create more disappointment. I didn't know how to process the resultant pain as it continued to fuel the anger and resentment building inside me.

Although I was sensitive by nature, there was also a side of me that was fiercely independent and determined to make my mark in the world. Not surprisingly, this was not acceptable to my father. His expectations of me were that I obeyed his rules without question as I followed in his footsteps.

His desire was for me to marry a farmer and give him lots of grandchildren. As I got older and bolder, I made no attempt to support this pretense. But my rebellion only made him more determined to break my spirit, forcing me to acquiesce to his demands. In his world, it was his way or the highway and anyone who dared challenge him was put at risk.

Our home was a war zone where yelling and hitting were everyday occurrences. But even in that environment, the sensitive me that loved my father was frightened that, in his eyes, I would never be good enough. It created in me an insecurity that believed people would look down on me if I didn't measure up to their expectations. When the sensitive me was in the driver's seat, the fierce, independent me would rise up and criticize her for being weak. This became my pattern for dealing with fear.

As my fears and insecurities grew, stress continued to build in my system. This unaddressed stress began to rise and I began to rail against the world, becoming angry and controlling, following in my father's footsteps, just as he had planned. Any laughter or joy that passed through my life was overshadowed by the anger and resentment that seethed inside me. I believed life wasn't worth living and death might be my only way out. But it wasn't until I was diagnosed with cancer for the third time that I woke up and realized that what we believe and perceive about ourselves creates our experience.

Outwardly I believed that no matter what others said or did to me, I could handle it. But deep inside, I suffered from self-loathing and low self-esteem. My experiences constantly reinforced that to make it in life, it was in my best interest to be subservient to men. I was convinced that my survival depended on it. I learned the hard way that when I didn't play by other people's rules, they could be cruel. And I learned that being anything other than what people wanted me to be was a recipe for disaster.

As I continued down this path, my heart began to shut down and I became critical, defensive, cynical and jealous of those who appeared to have a better life than mine. Day after day, I would rail against the injustices in the world and when someone hurt me, I never forgave or forgot!

On the inside I suffered, feeling guilty for my actions. This gave my ego plenty of ammunition to use my guilt as a weapon to heap shame on myself. To deal with this, I projected my guilt and shame onto others, convincing myself that "next time" I would do better. But doing better never came, creating a vicious cycle that strengthened my belief that I was a bad person, powerless to change.

I created unhealthy ways of coping. I embellished the truth in order to feel important. Believing it was impossible for me to have what I wanted simply by asking for it, I manipulated people into giving me what I wanted. When I did something wrong, I lied about it.

To add insult to injury, I lived in denial. But you can only perpetuate that ruse for so long before it turns on you. In an ironic twist, denial gives power to the very things we deny. While it may seem counterintuitive, the denied parts of the self end up running our lives. As I kept my negative beliefs and behaviors alive, they in turn impacted every choice and decision I made.

When we forget we are inherently good and instead take on the belief that there is something wrong with us, we become hostile and angry. We live a life we perceive as lacking in every way. Living in this mindset was devastating. Not only did I lack the things I so desperately wanted, like financial security and loving relationships, I also lacked compassion and joy. Since my role models had demonstrated lack in their lives, it was only natural I did the same. The consequence of living this way took its toll on me physically, emotionally and spiritually. I was unable to taste the sweetness of life and unable to feel any joy in my being.

As you can imagine, my brothers had their share of problems too. But for us, instead of coming together and protecting each other, we competed for every ounce of love we could get from our parents. This set the stage for pain and jealousy to define our relationships with each other. There was no place this was more evident than in school.

It is no surprise that since I was negative and toxic, I attracted people and experiences that were the same. In school, my classmates either ignored me or teased me mercilessly. It was a painful reminder of my perceived inadequacies, but what hurt the most was my brothers turning a blind eye to the dynamic, leaving me to fend for myself. I learned the hard way there was no one in my life I could trust or depend on, with one exception—my grandmother. She was the only person in my life who was there for me no matter what, the only person who truly loved and understood me. Time spent with her was the only time I felt completely safe.

After her death, when I was eighteen, I withdrew into a dark place. The use of alcohol became my chosen way to escape the pain. When that didn't prove strong enough, I used marijuana to numb me further. When these methods ran their course, I began to think that suicide might be the answer. That way, I reasoned, I would not only be free of pain, but free to join my grandmother as well.

Years later, once again facing my mortality, I realized my death wish was still alive and well. I also realized I had a choice: I could die bitter and lonely, or I could begin to really look at my destructive patterns and negative beliefs. Maybe I could even heal the cancer that was threatening my life for the third time. Plagued by constant thoughts of suicide, I was finally ready to accept the possibility that there might be a connection between the stress that was straining my system and the recurrence of my illness.

You may be asking what any of this has to do with a diagnosis of cancer. Research reveals that all illness is impacted by the unattended stress brought on by our thoughts, beliefs, and behaviors. Dr. Bruce Lipton, author of *The Biology of Belief*, says that positive, uplifting thoughts awaken and enliven our cells and the genes that produce a strong, healthy immune system. It follows then, that negative thoughts of any kind affect our cells and the genes that shut down our immune response. This in turn cripples our system's ability to cope with invaders that can lead to a compromised immune system, which eventually can lead to illness and disease.

From very early on my immune system was compromised. I can barely remember a time when I wasn't sick with something. Growing up in the stress of a hostile environment and taking on a pattern of negative behaviors lowered my system's ability to respond. My immune function was further impacted by the environmental toxins that came with growing up on a farm where pesticides and herbicides were used to grow crops. Being exposed to these contaminants on a daily basis and living downwind from Hanford, a nuclear facility that had leaked radiation into the air during the fifties, made my body vulnerable. I was unable to handle the daily toxic assault.

Around the age of twelve, I began suffering from a series of sinus, ear, and bladder infections that kept me home from school for days at a time. After multiple trips to doctors and months of being sick, I started to believe there was no cure for what ailed me. This served to reinforce my core belief that there was something inherently wrong with me.

Over the next several years, the struggle continued. But I kept my eye on the future, convinced that graduating from high school, leaving home, and making my way in the world was not only going to change my circumstances, but magically release me from my problems. However, as I would soon learn, my well-laid plans were not meant to be. Instead of heading down the road to success and happiness, I was headed down the slippery slope of more pain and struggle. A life that would look suspiciously similar to my childhood!

2

I Married My Father

Relationships are our greatest teachers. It is through our relationships that our wounded self is reflected back to us, and why our most intimate connections produce our most powerful lessons. I was about to experience this truth in a big way.

When Bob appeared at my apartment with a friend of mine, he knocked me off my feet. He was clearly a catch—handsome, smart, well-dressed, and slick as the red Pontiac he drove. He was also the first man to ever give me chills.

Day after day, I fantasized about having him as my boyfriend. Over the next several months, he came in and out of my life, flirting with me every time our paths crossed. Then one day, to my complete surprise, he asked me out on a date. I was in heaven. The man of my dreams was showing interest in me, a young girl with stars in her eyes and love on her mind. But right from the start there were warning signs and red flags I refused to see.

Our first date ended in an argument. He was opinionated, dominating and needed to be right. Maybe if I'd been paying attention instead of being enthralled with his good looks and sex appeal, I would have recognized this pattern. I might have recognized my father in him. But I was too caught up in the heat of our connection to notice that he constantly badgered me. He didn't approve of the people I spent time with. He criticized the way I dressed, telling me my clothes were too sexy and this was the reason men were attracted to me. I didn't see anything wrong with the way I dressed but his constant criticism evoked an old pattern in me—do anything to make him happy. That's what mattered. Gradually, I caved. I began to dress the way he wanted, all the while convincing myself he was right, maybe I was getting too much attention. What motivated my decision to comply with his demands was something my mother taught me: when you're with a man, you are his to do with what he wants.

As our relationship progressed, I found myself saying yes to him when I really meant no. He wanted me with him all the time. Whatever he was doing, he wanted me there. I was flattered to think he needed me. Flattered that he loved me so much he couldn't bear to be away from me. He was a hunter—a sport I could not stomach–but he needed me. Hunting wasn't the same without me. So while a voice deep inside was telling me the real reason he wanted me was because he didn't trust me to be on my own, I ignored it. I wasn't able to trust that voice and submerged my feelings, acquiescing to his demands.

Progressively, he insisted I spend less time with my friends and more time with him. Soon, I found myself agreeing to all his demands, reasoning it was easier to simply "go along" than to argue. As the days became weeks and the weeks became months, saying yes became my primary means of pleasing him, thus avoiding an argument. "No" became a word I dropped from my vocabulary.

The more this dysfunction became a part of my everyday life, the more I felt compelled to ask permission to do even the simplest things. Simultaneously, a battle raged within between the part of me that knew this wasn't right and the part of me that was trained to obey the man in my life. As I stuffed my feelings, quieting the part of me that knew better, I willingly gave him more and more power over me. Finally, and insidiously, he was in complete control of our relationship and me. So convinced that making him happy was far more important than making me happy, my motto became "Anything to please him."

Out of touch with my own needs and wants, I found myself in a relationship with a man exactly like my father. But instead of running the other direction, I married him. I entered into a marriage with the hope that someday he'd change and we'd live happily ever after–but he had other plans.

When we first met, I was living in a city where I wanted to settle down. But immediately after the wedding, we moved into a little house in a small community next to the Canadian border. Before I knew what hit me, I was stranded in the middle of nowhere living with a man I didn't know. Rather than speak up, I kept silent, hoping things would change. Years of conditioning had taught me to be a good wife.

And to be a good wife, you let your husband make the important decisions. After all, I was eighteen, married to a handsome prince, with my whole life ahead of me. I was so lucky—he could have had anyone.

Within six months, with him gone most of the time running a small business, I was home alone, living in a house across the road from his interfering parents. My romantic fantasy of happily ever after was nowhere to be found. On weekends, neither was he. He spent Friday and Saturday nights at the local bar with his best friend while I remained home alone to ponder the question, "What the hell have I gotten myself into?"

After two years of fighting with him and his parents, our marriage began to unravel. That's when I finally got the courage to threaten him with divorce if we didn't move back to the city where we could make a life together. He was very resistant to the idea, but having found part of my voice, I kept at him.

One night, driving home drunk at a high rate of speed, he slammed into a herd of cows crossing the road, killing one and totaling his car. Luckily he wasn't seriously hurt, but he was enraged with me, saying my constant nagging and complaining caused him to go off the deep end. I was the reason he was drunk and driving recklessly.

What happened after the accident came as a shock to both of us. His father, after hearing the excuse Bob was using for his reckless behavior, told his son it was time to grow up and do what needed to be done to save his marriage. Bob, side-swiped by his father's reaction, decided maybe moving to the city was the best thing. This was a tremendous relief to me. Not only did it give me what I wanted but it also absolved me of having to carry out my threat of divorce. In spite of believing that leaving Bob was the right thing to do, I wasn't sure I could follow through with it.

Over the next few months, things started to look up. Bob was able to find a buyer for his business and we found a perfect house in the city. For the first time since our wedding, I had hope that things would fall into place. My hopes were short-lived.

"I hate it here. It's nothing but cement and more cement," he complained. "Chalk up another lame move by Brenda!"

Being reminded on a daily basis that I was the reason his life was a mess, I started to believe him. To deal with the pain, I denied my feelings, pushing away the guilt that consumed me. Instead, I put all my time and energy into getting a job. After a two-month search,

I landed one as a receptionist with a top mortgage company in town. In the meantime, Bob found a job as a laborer, giving him something else to hate about living in the city. But I forged on, thinking that in time he'd realize we were better off living in a place where we could meet new friends and create a life.

As my denial of the situation deepened, causing me to emotionally detach and withhold sex, his discontent and resentment of me continued to fester. Increasingly, the verbal and physical abuse became more threatening, until one Christmas when it reached a zenith.

It was one of those beautiful, crisp, cold days when the sky was the kind of blue you get lost in. As I drove home from the office singing Christmas carols, I imagined Bob's pride in me when he learned I had earned a large cash bonus. And along with the cash, a set of sterling silver-rimmed drinking glasses. I was so excited to share my bounty!

As usual, Bob arrived home before I did and buried himself in a six-pack of beer. I wasn't surprised to see empty bottles on the table. What did surprise me was his reaction when I handed him my check and showed him the glasses.

Looking up, he sneered at me. "What's this about? What'd you do to earn this, sleep with your boss?"

Shocked at his accusation, I went into defense mode. "No, no, not at all! It's just that our company had one of its best years yet and management wanted to thank all of us for doing such a good job."

But he wasn't interested in my explanation and continued with his accusations. As things intensified, a screaming match ensued and he smashed two glasses into the fireplace.

"Get these goddamn things out of my sight or I'll crush the rest of them!"

Something snapped inside me. "Go to hell!!!" I screamed.

That's when he jumped off the couch, pinned my hands behind my back, and pushed me to the floor. Desperate to stop his assault, I agreed, "Fine. I'll get rid of the glasses. I'll get rid of them."

"And stop banging your boss?" he yelled an inch from my face.

"There is nothing going on with my boss," I cried. "Nothing!"

"You're a liar. Always have been, always will be!" he zeroed in, continuing to press me to the floor.

Suddenly it hit me. He wasn't interested in the truth, he was interested in hurting me. He wanted to shame me into saying what he wanted to hear. He didn't even care if I had actually done the deed he was accusing me of. He believed I had and he wasn't going to stop hurting me until I admitted it.

As he continued to press his knee into my chest, making it almost impossible for me to breathe, I finally gave him what he wanted. "Alright," I crumbled. "Yes, it's true. What you say is true."

A look of triumph came over his face and he jumped up and ran out the door.

As he drove off, I lay there thinking it would only be a matter of time before he really hurt me. But my fear of being alone, of not being able to support myself, outweighed my instincts. Cleaning up the mess, I vowed that next time, I'd say whatever he wanted me to say. That, I prayed, might be the way to curb his violence.

My job became my sanctuary. I was living a double life. Bob's constant suspicions and forced isolations were an ongoing threat to my wellbeing. The only reason he allowed me to work was because we needed the money. In an effort to keep him from making me quit, I never talked about work or let my coworkers into my private life. To keep them from becoming suspicious about my repeated requests that they not call me at home, I made the excuse that Bob needed quiet time because of his stressful job. The truth was, I knew he could combust at any moment.

A call one day from my best friend at work who was facing a small emergency set the stage for one of those moments. I could hear the desperation in her voice and knew I needed to speak with her. I was also acutely aware of Bob's displeasure that someone would call me at home and did my best to keep our conversation short.

Once off the phone, I turned to make my way outside, thinking he might be less inclined to start something in front of our neighbors. But he was on to me, and just as I was about to step outside, he grabbed me from behind pulling me back into the house, screaming obscenities at me. Desperate to save myself and stop his attack, I apologized profusely, swearing it would never happen again. But in my heart I knew it was only a matter of time before something else would set him off. Unable to get a handle on this crippling fear, I stayed, convincing myself I had no choice.

If I had understood the influence of my dysfunctional role models, I wouldn't have needed to look very far for answers. I married out of need and desperation, looking for someone to complete me. I didn't have a clue what a real partnership was. I wanted respect, cooperation, and mutual support, but instead I found a competitive ego that constantly battled me for the upper hand. I was physically a grown woman but psychologically still a frightened little girl trying to please her father. Only this time my father was disguised as my husband.

A lifetime of feeling unworthy of loving relationships created a scenario that brought pain and destruction. My negative beliefs had me convinced I couldn't have a man in my life that treated me with the respect I craved. I proved my hypothesis by attracting a man who tried to control me. The result was a viscous cycle of negativity that poisoned our marriage and made us both miserable.

Living this way on a daily basis, my body started its decline. In a déjà vu of my childhood, I began to manifest one physical problem after another: recurring bladder and yeast infections that lasted for months; colds and flus that turned into ear infections and infected tonsils that kept me on antibiotics for weeks. I didn't realize the drugs, coupled with the stress, would have long-term effects on my health, nor did I realize the illnesses plaguing me were red flags of a more serious condition I was not willing to see, let alone take responsibility for. All I could see was me, trapped in a marriage with no way out, the victim of a man who was the cause of all my problems. Then one day, fate intervened. The wars raging within me, one with my husband and one with myself, finally converged.

3

Diagnosis and Recovery

With my twenty-sixth birthday approaching and Bob and I celebrating our eighth anniversary, I was given a diagnosis of cervical cancer. At the time I was in so much mental torment and emotional pain that when the doctors told me what they had discovered, part of me felt relieved. I was so desperate, I thought having cancer might be the impetus to turn our marriage around, to bring Bob to his senses and force him to change. I believed cancer could be the solution to our problems. What I failed to consider was that it was *my* body in crisis, not his.

In dealing with my illness, I simply did what I had been taught. I put myself in the hands of modern medicine, relinquishing all decisions to my doctors. Educating myself about alternative options was not even in my consciousness. And the concept of looking at the cancer as a symptom of something bigger in my life, well let's just say that was beyond my scope. All I wanted was to get my marriage back on track, release my emotional pain, and get rid of the cancer.

My doctors recommended a hysterectomy, which would eliminate the possibility of ever having children. Bob and I had never discussed having children. However, before the diagnosis I had a choice; now, that choice was being taken away. Unable to take in the seriousness of what I was facing or talk with Bob about my feelings, let alone talk about his, I chose denial. The pain in my marriage overrode everything, including the seriousness of my diagnosis or the consequences of a hysterectomy.

I made the decision to go ahead with the surgery. After all, having children would only complicate things between us. At the consultation with my doctor I lied, telling him Bob and I had discussed it and were in agreement. Confused and scared, I was unable to comprehend the weight of my solo decision on my future or the future of our marriage.

When it came time for surgery, I was consumed with fear. Even though my parents and Bob were present, my inability to trust anyone left me feeling alone and isolated. I compensated for this lack of trust by convincing myself I didn't need anyone—I could handle whatever came along. I needed to protect myself from depending on others. I had experienced enough disappointment for a lifetime!

Settled in my room, my parents did their best to make small talk with Bob while I stared out the window, avoiding the tension between them. My parents weren't fond of him. My dad had been particularly skeptical about our marriage lasting, and while my mother pretended to be okay with our relationship, she too had her doubts. Now, at a time when I longed for us to come together, the chasm only seemed to widen.

It wasn't that they thought Bob was a bad person. They just never warmed to him. He was difficult to talk to and not much for socializing. Maybe they sensed something wasn't right between us. If they did, they never let on. And as with everything, they didn't ask questions and I in turn kept my opinions to myself.

After several uncomfortable minutes of increasing strain, a nurse finally showed up. I needed someone in my corner and had high hopes she would be that sensitive presence. Unfortunately, she was cold and intimidating, approaching her work as though it were a chore she could barely tolerate. And though it wasn't the support I was hoping for, a part of me could relate. Her behavior reminded me of how I felt about my job.

Though I loved the people I worked with, I wasn't in love with the mortgage business. My job merely served to pay bills and allowed me a short respite from my relationship. As I watched her take my vital signs, I wondered if she was escaping some painful circumstances in her life. This perspective helped me to accept her, even though she wasn't what I had hoped for.

Throughout my stay, she continued to be cold and distant while I continued to excuse her behavior, thinking we shared some kind of painful bond. At times I felt the urge to speak up, but didn't. I knew no one likes a complainer so I suffered in silence, "happy face" firmly in place. Meanwhile, I deluded myself into believing I could handle what was happening to me. That having cancer and a hysterectomy at twenty-six was no big deal.

It was impossible for me to see my illness as a warning sign. A warning sign that my life was out of balance, that my body was trying to get my attention. With no role models who perceived illness as a possible messenger of deeper issues, I remained unaware that my body might be trying to tell me something. I didn't know it would continue to give me messages until I was ready to take responsibility for my life.

Surgery is an extremely stressful shock to the body. Being so out of touch with mine, I was unable to have compassion for what I was going through. I was young. I expected a lot of myself. I had no patience for what I perceived as weakness. My heart was shut down, closed for business, unaware that without an open channel there could be no compassion. But opening the heart is risky business. It requires vulnerability, something I was not very good at. It was easier for me to let my mind be in charge. It was also why, when things didn't go as planned, I felt angry and bitter, buying into the old adage my dad used to spout, "Life is a struggle and then you die."

Once home from the hospital, I started experiencing hot flashes and rapid mood changes. Crying jags became a daily occurrence. Day after day I woke up feeling irritated and exhausted while Bob did his best to ignore me. One day, having reached the end of his rope, he started in on me.

"So, Brenda, are we ever going to have sex again?"

Hoping this was idle chatter, I continued on my way as if I hadn't heard him.

"Brenda?" he bellowed. "Are you going deaf now, too?"

I stopped. "What?" I inquired. "Did you say something?"

"Sex," he articulated. "Are we ever going to have it again?"

"Well, Bob," I started. "You know the doctor said we need to wait at least three months."

"You are something!" he raged. "What are you gonna do when you run out of excuses?"

"It's not an excuse," I reasoned. "I had a major surgery and . . . "

"I know what you had, Brenda," he interrupted. "I was there, remember?"

"I know, Bob. I know you were there. I'm not saying you . . . "

"What are you saying?" he asked with the smirk I'd come to recognize all too well.

"Look," I said, eager to put an end to this line of questioning and restore peace, a rare commodity in our home. "I'll ask. My next doctor visit, I'll ask him about it."

I knew full well what he would say but for a short time this seemed to appease Bob. That is until his next urge. Exhausted and tired of fighting about it, I called my doctor and asked him to speak to Bob. I had no idea what a mistake that would turn out to be. Bob, not hearing what he wanted to hear from the doctor, became enraged.

Hanging up the phone, he said, "That's it. We're doing it and we're doing it now!"

Every cell of my body shut down and another piece of me died. I knew he would not take no for an answer. And despite what my body and soul were telling me, keeping the peace took over and I acquiesced.

During my next two check-ups I held my breath as the doctor examined me, hoping he wouldn't notice that Bob and I had had intercourse. Thankfully he didn't. But even if he had and insisted we refrain, I would have disobeyed him. I knew I was in far greater danger from saying no to Bob than from disobeying my doctor's orders.

The following months were hell as I struggled with exhaustion and the discomfort from repeated intercourse. On my days off work, I used television and fantasy books to numb my pain. At work I wore my smiley face pretending my marriage was fine and I was great.

During subsequent checks with the doctor I longed to confide in him but my fear of Bob's reprisal and the shame I felt about lying to the doctor stopped me from reaching out. Six months had passed since my surgery and although my tests indicated I was doing well, I continued to feel depressed and fatigued. It was during this period that I first thought perhaps it wasn't the surgery but rather the stress of my living situation that was the culprit.

"Bob," I started. "I know things have been kind of difficult around here and . . . "

"Really? I hadn't noticed." That smirk again.

I continued, ignoring the fire in my belly. "I was thinking that we might benefit from therapy."

"What?" he said, screwing up his face in disbelief.

"Therapy," I tried again. "Couples therapy."

"What the f . . . ." Shaking his head, he stood, looked at me in total disgust and started to leave the room.

Part of me was relieved. "Well, that's that," I thought. "At least I tried. I should get some points for that, shouldn't I?" But then, just as abruptly as he had turned on his heels to leave, he spun around and came back.

"What the hell is the matter with you, Brenda? Therapy? Are you actually serious or is this more of your delusion?"

"I just thought, Bob . . . "

"Well, see there? There's your problem, Brenda. Stop it. Stop thinking. You don't do it very well. I don't need therapy. Therapy is for losers, Brenda. Maybe that's why you're so eager to go."

I stood steadfast, girding myself not to cry. I would not let him see me weak. I would not give him another inch of my self-respect.

"I am insulted you would even bring it up," he continued. "Clearly someone around here has problems but it sure as hell ain't me. So, Brenda, you wanna go to therapy, go with my blessings. Let the therapist tell you you're an overreacting lunatic. My relationship is just fine. If yours isn't working out, that's your problem. Don't make it mine."

Dumbfounded by his response, it was clear to me I had two choices. I could change, or leave. But even in the light of his latest tirade, the thought of leaving, living on my own, was still more terrifying than staying in my marriage. So instead of continuing to campaign for counseling, I waited. I waited for just the right moment to make my move, praying I would have the courage to do what needed to be done.

Not long after our "talk," we had another horrible episode. Often our fights were merely shouting matches where words were the weapons we used to hurt one another. But for the second time in a month our fighting took a disturbing turn. There was the usual screaming and Bob pushing me up against a wall, but this time there was a fierceness in his eyes I hadn't seen before. A determination that communicated to me I was in real danger.

In light of this episode, an interesting thing happened. The same part of me that was aware I was in danger took control over my being. I didn't yell or scream at Bob, nor did I try to run. This time I stood my ground, allowing Bob to do "his thing." Then, I walked away knowing this was the last time I would have to endure his anger and rage. The choice before me was suddenly crystal clear. I was done.

The following day, after Bob went to work, I gathered my things and walked out the door. I had an epiphany that day: I had been living his life, not mine. I had only friends he approved of, wore clothes he thought appropriate, participated in hobbies and sports only if he could participate with me, and put up with his verbal, emotional, and physical abuse. I had allowed myself to be beaten down so far I had no idea who I was. Now, for the first time in twelve years I was ready to put it all behind me. I gathered what was left of my self-esteem, promising myself I would never again allow any man to treat me the way Bob had.

Having worked up the courage to leave, I experienced a short period of euphoria when my confidence was at an all-time high. I had done the right thing. However, my high didn't last long. Fear soon crept into the recesses of my mind and started spewing all the reasons I should have stayed. Top of the list was that Bob, despite his flaws, could be a really good guy. Yes, he had a temper and was sometimes cruel. But, like my father, he also had the ability to be kind and loving when he wanted to. I was beginning to understand what might have kept my mother in her marriage. As these thoughts took hold, I started to question whether walking out had been a mistake.

With few friends to lean on, I found myself alone and slipping deeper and deeper into self-doubt. Worry was my constant state of being. My parents worried, too. They felt I had made a hasty decision leaving Bob without a plan in place. They were concerned I might not be able to support myself, which only fed my own insecurities about what I had done. At work I was unable to concentrate or be productive and was in danger of losing my job.

To add fire to this scenario, friends informed me Bob was going out almost every night carousing with women, living the high life. It infuriated me to know that as I sat locked in my tiny apartment barely able to pay my bills, Bob was living it up while he lived in "our" house without a moment's discontent.

When I looked honestly at my reality, I had to admit my parents were right. I had left Bob without a plan in place. And painful as it was, I had to admit the man I loved, the man I thought had my best interests at heart, had no intention of playing fair. Consequently, I ended up with my car (and the payments), my clothes, and my portable TV, a gift from my parents. Bob, on the other hand, absconded with everything else, including our furniture.

Alone and angry with myself for marrying him, I was once again living out the consequences of my belief that there must be something wrong with me. Why else would this be happening?

As the months dragged on and I continued to struggle at work, I was put on probation. My resentment, now at an all-time high, was reflected in my inability to get along with anyone in my life. Feelings of hopelessness began to shape everything while my issues and problems continued to play out. In an attempt to dull my pain I turned to alcohol, marijuana, and indiscriminate sex.

Night after night I found myself in a different bar—cigarette in hand—ready to go home with anyone who caught my attention. My grand scheme was that eventually word would get back to Bob that I was sleeping around and he'd feel the same pain I was feeling. With only revenge on my mind, I never realized I was the only person being hurt by my behavior.

As the weeks blurred one into another, I witnessed my life going downhill at breakneck speed. Little did I know that by focusing on everything wrong in my life, I was setting in motion another life-threatening crisis; a crisis that this time, no one could have imagined. Least of all me.

Part Two

Illness as a Teacher

4

A Familiar Sadness

As the months wore on I plummeted ever deeper into my dysfunction. I continued to drink heavily, smoke, get stoned and have promiscuous unprotected sex. One morning waking from a binge, a long forgotten feeling came over me and I felt compelled to pray; something I hadn't done since my childhood church days.

Typically in prayer we plead with God to save us, expecting Him to perform a miracle, plucking us from peril. But God doesn't work that way. God works *through* us, not apart from us. To benefit from His power we must be in a state of surrender and acceptance. Only in that consciousness, in the sacred place where God is present can He work through us helping to transform our lives.

I know what you must be thinking. Why didn't I take my own advice? The answer is easy. At the time I had no clue how to connect to this powerful loving energy. It was later on my journey that I learned the merits of transformative prayer. Later when the bottom had already fallen out. Later when I was finally able to surrender the will of my ego and accept God's will for me instead. And not until later, in this place of surrender and acceptance that I was open enough for this higher wisdom to make itself known.

This is one of the gifts of adversity. It pushes us to a crisis point where we have to make a choice—surrender and change, or continue suffering. When adversity shows up as a life-threatening disease, the choice is even more pressing—surrender and change, or face possible death. Not that the act of surrender and change guarantees you will survive a life-threatening disease. What it does guarantee is that while you're in physical form you have the opportunity to come to a place of deep peace and joy. For many, that alone can help save a life.

This feeling of peace and joy was something I desperately wanted in my life. But I was a lost soul filled with anger and despair, clueless about how to experience these feelings. One day during one of my plentiful pity parties I caught a glimpse of myself in a mirror. Staring back at me was someone I didn't recognize. Her skin was gray and lined, her body malnourished and emaciated. As I moved my gaze to her eyes, I saw something I could no longer deny—a deep familiar sadness that until that moment I hadn't allowed myself to see.

Jolted by this vision, shame engulfed me. Followed by the all too familiar voice, "Look at you! You're a mess! You'll never amount to anything!" Unable to deny what I was hearing and seeing, I fell to the floor, sobbing until I cried myself to sleep. When I awoke a few hours later I was surprised to find I felt better. Momentarily striped of all my defenses, a picture began forming in my mind—me, moving away to someplace new, a place where no one knew me. I could leave my past behind and start over.

"Could it really be that simple?" I asked myself. "Yes" was the answer I heard. "Wow! Why didn't I think of this sooner?"

This is how it happens. One minute you're miserable and scared, the next your mind is offering an instant solution that feels like you've just been given the keys to the kingdom. But here's the rub. That familiar voice I heard, the voice I had been mistakenly using as my guide was the voice of my ego self, not the voice of my higher self. How did I know that? I didn't until much later when I began to awaken and distinguish between the two.

I now understand it takes experience to discern the difference between guidance by spirit and guidance by ego. The truth is until we connect to spirit or higher power, the voice we hear will invariably be that of the ego. What's confounding about this voice is that it presents itself as the voice that has the answers to all our problems. In truth it does not. The ego is self-serving, concerned with its own agenda and loves being right. Given the opportunity the ego will choose being right over being happy every time. The ego is also skilled at making us believe it has the answer to everything. Offering up solutions that are embedded in the illusion of a quick fix and instant gratification.

In contrast, the voice of the higher self comes from deep within and can only be heard when one is quiet, calm and receptive. Being aware of God's presence requires that we slow down and focus on connecting with this loving energy merely for the sake of connection and nothing more. Sitting quietly in nature, breathing or meditating, all serve to create this connection. Once hooked in, you will be guided to the answers you seek as long as you are willing to trust what is being given. When you hear the whisper of the divine you can trust the message is coming from the most compassionate loving part of yourself. Originating in that glorious part of your soul where forgiveness, humility, charity and grace are found.

By contrast, the ego looks for solutions in the material world using whomever or whatever it needs to reach its desired goal. It uses fear and urgency to motivate us to react and respond to its immediate needs. One of the many fears my ego used was to convince me my life was never going to change, that suffering and struggle would always define me. Now, in the wake of the pain I was feeling, my ego was offering me a quick fix, an easy solution—move away, start over, leave my past behind. My ego mind made it sound as though this was the perfect solution to my problems. I was the queen of running away. I had this covered!

The ego's rhetoric can be very seductive. And I was not immune. The very next day I marched into my office and asked my manager for a transfer to our Seattle office. Getting transferred would relieve me of finding another job. Plus, having a ready-made job would definitely make my case for moving. How could anyone question my motives?

Soon after putting my request in for a transfer, it was granted. I couldn't believe my luck. Things were looking up already. With that settled, I needed to find a place to live. As I was hatching my plan I happened to run into a friend who was also looking to relocate to Seattle. We decided to get an apartment together. The following weekend we made our way to Seattle and found the perfect place to live.

With my life finally falling into place, I needed to move to the next phase of my plan, financing my move and immediate living expenses. My parents were the likely candidates but I knew it wasn't going to be easy. They were old-fashioned and didn't believe in making life changes until a good solid plan was in place. Unfortunately I hadn't thought to present them with a reasonable plan. So when they turned me down, though I was disappointed I knew I couldn't let my feelings get in the way. I buried the hurt and got to work on a plan that was certain to get them onboard.

A few weeks later, having done my research, I showed them a list of housing prices in Spokane and Seattle. This comparison would prove to them the Northwest market was a better place for me to make money. I pointed out, now that I was a loan officer dependent on sales to make a living, relocating to Seattle was the right move for me. After much discussion and evaluation they agreed.

With them now in my corner my campaign for financial assistance kicked into full gear. After four weeks of dropping hints about my unstable financial position and the fact that it could take up to six months for me to see a paycheck, they capitulated offering to pay my moving expenses and first month's rent. With all my ducks in a row I was on my way to a brand-new life.

Once settled in our apartment, my roomie and I decided to meet the neighborhood. We dressed in our sexiest outfits and cruised down to the hottest bar in town to check things out. Exiting my marriage, I had been terrified of being single again. But I quickly found I loved being on my own. Not only was no one telling me what to do but I was also receiving positive attention from men. Attention I had so futilely craved from Bob.

He had no trouble fawning over his women friends and co-workers, well aware of the pain this caused me, like being stabbed in the heart. But he continued this behavior because he wanted to make sure I knew how lucky I was he had chosen me. This was one of the ways he exercised control and because I was insecure and afraid to be alone, I was the perfect target.

Fridays quickly became girls' night out. One night around midnight my friends and I ended up in one of our favorite haunts. As we waltzed through the door my radar was up, scanning the room for available guys. That's when I spotted him, a gorgeous specimen sitting at the bar. Like a laser beam I zeroed in. It didn't take long to get his attention. As our eyes locked, tingling sensations shot down my spine. And when he came over to talk to me, well, let's just say he had me at "Hello!"

I learned he was the co-owner of a small construction company that was in the middle of securing finances for a new project. Jackpot! Not only was he gorgeous, but down the road he would be good for my business. A few drinks later he told me he had recently divorced his wife and was looking to have a good time. Since having a good time was at the top of my agenda, this felt like a match made in heaven. We made plans to get together again.

Once home, away from his good looks and charming ways I found myself reconsidering a subsequent get-together. When it came to men, trust was a big hill to climb. As I pondered how to get out of it I heard, "What are you thinking? You just met Prince Charming and you want to let him go? What if he meets someone else? That would be a tragedy." As my thoughts turned to fear, I put my trust issues on the back burner deciding I'd better pursue this relationship now. If I didn't, I might regret it.

When we met up a few days later I was pleasantly surprised to find that Scott, my Prince Charming, had a magical quality to him. Our communication came so easily. For the first time, I felt safe and comfortable to be myself around a man. Over the course of the next few months as he continued to earn my trust, our relationship deepened.

My dream in life had been to become an actress and model, a dream no one knew. But I wanted Scott to know. I longed to have the man in my life support me in pursuing my goals. His encouragement gave me the boost I needed and not long after telling him my secret, I signed up for acting and modeling classes.

Acting came very naturally to me and quickly became one of my favorite things to do. That is until one night when I was doing a scene in class and my acting coach made a derogatory remark that sent me into a downward spiral. It brought back all the criticism I got from my father and Bob. Old memories and emotional baggage I had suppressed over the years emerged with a vengeance.

I was instantly ten again, a time when my dreams of becoming an actress and model had become very real to me. Every chance I got I studied pictures of models in magazines. Alone in my room I would stand in front of the mirror emulating poses and mimicking actresses I saw on television. When no one was around, the kitchen became my Paris runway where I would refine my walk preparing for the fairytale life I was sure I would lead.

One afternoon while helping my father clean the shop my mind flitted from walking the runways in Paris to Oscar night where I would receive my Academy Award. As my thoughts drifted, I wanted desperately to share them with my father. I wanted his attention and more than anything, to include him in my world beyond the farm. Lost in my fantasies, I made the mistake of forgetting he already had a plan for me. As far as he was concerned I was going to college and that was that.

As I babbled on unaware of his agitation, he abruptly turned on his heels and stomped toward the house shaking his head as he always did when he was disappointed in me. Mortified I froze in place while the voice in my head criticized me for being so stupid. I learned a painful lesson that day. Never tell anyone your dreams, especially your family.

Scott, of course had no idea of my experience that night in class. Confused about my quitting after my initial excitement, he wanted to know why. In tears, I confessed what had happened and the memory of my father that had surfaced.

"Oh, Brenda," he said, love filling his eyes, "can you see that this is a huge turning point for you?"

I wanted to see but I was too filled with my own shame, my own sense of disappointment that I would never live up to my own expectations . . . or my father's.

"Can you see," he went on, "you have a choice?"

"But I've chosen so many times before and it never turns out the way I want."

"How long are you going to let others decide your fate? When will it be time to go for what you want?"

While I understood the sense of what he was saying, it didn't ease my pain or quell the awareness I now had that when my father walked away that day, the little girl in me who believed the world was her oyster had died. She had been replaced by someone who over time, not only lost her confidence but was perpetually terrified of being rejected.

While it's not unusual for fear to surface when one is about to embark on something new, once thoughts and beliefs that support this fear begin to take hold, confidence is lost. The mind begins to build stories that substantiate this doubt and fear. As a consequence of that experience with my father, my mind made up several stories, stories I began to believe. I was carrying a lot of destructive baggage that was keeping me from reaching out and making my dreams come true. Now with a loving partner, one that believed in me, I was being given the opportunity to move past my fears. Was it actually possible I could heal the baggage that for years had kept me from pursuing what I really wanted?

With Scott's support and a willingness to process some of my painful emotions, I got back on the road to making my dreams a reality. At the same time, my nighttime dreams took me by surprise. In these dreams I was standing in front of television cameras talking to a live audience hosting some kind of talk show. While it was exciting to think I might be destined for a life in front of the camera, it was not what my daydreams had been made of. My love was acting, not asking questions of guests on a television show. Nevertheless, this dream continued for the next several months.

Then one night after acting class, one of my classmates asked me to have a drink with her. The subject of nightmares and dreams came up and I told her about this dream I was having. She shared that her mother was taking a dream class and had learned that the dream state is where we process things we can't process during our waking hours. "Hmm," I thought, "is that what I'm doing?" Her mother also said dreams can be signs of things to come, good and bad. As soon as the words were out of her mouth a shiver went down my spine. With my luck I would probably be one of those people being warned of something bad about to happen.

On the drive home I couldn't shake the feeling. It was then that Scott's words echoed in the back of my mind, prompting me to ask myself, "Was I going to move forward or let someone else decide my fate?" Still shaken but determined to follow my heart, there was one thing of which I was sure. I did not want to live a life of regret.

5

Making Other Plans

At the same time, Scott was also at a turning point in his life, certain he didn't want to stay in the construction business. When I asked him what he was passionate about, he said he wasn't sure what he wanted to do but he knew he wanted to make a difference in the world. It seemed as though the time was ripe for us to make a move. We had talked before about turning our dreams into reality so, seizing the moment we made plans to marry and move to Los Angeles to pursue our dreams together.

Life was good—better than I ever imagined it could be. That's why when I discovered a lump on my breast I was shocked. Here I was about to be married to the love of my life, about to move to Los Angeles to pursue my dream, when suddenly everything was being threatened. Why was this happening to me? Claiming I was too busy planning my wedding, I ignored the problem. That is until the lump became so painful that I was forced to pay attention.

As reluctant as I was at first to see a doctor, I went on to seek a second and third opinion because deep inside a little voice kept insisting there was more to this than I was being told. Each doctor insisted it was nothing more than an infected milk gland and I was given a prescription for antibiotics and told to get on with my life. Granted, I had no logical basis for questioning my doctors' opinions, but the message I was receiving and the feelings it evoked were too strong to be denied.

I was awakening in new and unexpected ways and though I didn't know exactly what to do with these newfound feelings, I wanted desperately to make them mean something. However, I wasn't quite there yet. There was a deep part of me that was unsettled by the doctors' diagnosis but the conscious part of me was too steeped in fear to listen to my inner knowing.

It is always within our power to choose. We can allow the powerful energy of fear to motivate or to paralyze, to support us when crises occur or destroy us in the process. But I wasn't ready to listen fully to my inner voice. I was still the product of believing the experts knew best. If they said it was nothing, then I would go with that. I had a life to plan!

After the wedding, Scott sold his half of the business, I quit my job, and we moved to Los Angeles to start our new life together. Friends and family were happy for us although they couldn't seem to resist dropping hints that we might be making a mistake. We heard the rumblings.

"Moving to Los Angeles without jobs, what are they thinking?"

As for my father, he was in top form. "Brenda, what are you doing with your life?"

"Dad, I . . ."

"Just shut up and listen! Your grand plan is to quit a well-paying guaranteed job and go try to find a job, if you can call it a job, making believe? Is that it?"

"Dad, I . . ."

"Do you know who gets those jobs?"

"Well, there are . . . ."

"*Not* girls like you. Not middle-aged . . ."

"I'm not middle . . ."

"Not middle-aged farm girls like you. Those jobs go to young beautiful girls. What are you thinking?"

And so it went. But for the first time in my life, I had a man in my corner who believed in me. A man who shared my dream of living a life we loved. Armed with that belief in each other, we carried on, determined to follow our hearts and not allow my father or anyone else to stand in our way.

Once in LA, we executed our plan. I immediately enrolled in acting class while Scott set out to find work. I found a few modeling jobs to help make ends meet while Scott found work as a crew member in the film industry hoping it would lead to something bigger. Though it was a meager beginning, we were excited to be moving in the right direction. That's when the bomb dropped.

One day during a modeling job, my employer pulled me aside.

"Brenda, are you okay?" she inquired. "There's something missing. Something off. You're not your usually sparkly self. What is it?"

"I'm fine." I said, knowing I was anything but fine.

"Brenda?" she said, not believing a word of it.

"Well, I do have this . . ."

"What?"

"A lump," I whispered.

"What? A lump? Where?"

"My breast."

"Oh, Brenda. How long have you had it?" she asked with razor focus.

"It's actually been several months now," I said, now fully engulfed in embarrassment.

"Follow me," she said springing into action. She grabbed my wrist and pulled me to her office. Once there she found her address book, looked up a number, and dialed the phone.

"I'm calling my doctor and setting up an appointment for you . . . now!"

Well aware that her sister had recently died of breast cancer, I allowed her to intervene.

"This is the name and address of the doctor," she said writing it on a Post-it note. "Listen to me, Brenda," now zeroing in on me. "You can not deal with the beast you do not know. You need to get informed, find out what is going on with your body so you know how to handle it. Don't run from this, you'll only make it worse. Dr. K will take care of you. Go get informed and let me know what happens. You'll be fine."

With that she came around her desk, gave me a hug, and sent me on my way.

To that point I'd been fairly successful at keeping a lid on my fear, but after witnessing her reaction, I couldn't help but think I might be in deep trouble. Arriving home, I was in serious need of a hug. Unfortunately, it would have to wait. Scott was at work and restricted from receiving calls. Without my support system, my mind went spinning out of control.

As the evening wore on, my fear and panic escalated. I briefly thought about calling friends in Seattle. Hell, I even thought about calling my mom but quickly nixed that idea. If I called her I'd have to admit my parents had been right. Leaving Seattle with no money and no support was not only shortsighted but also foolish.

That night I couldn't sleep, nor could I stop my mind from offering up one dark scenario after another. When Scott finally got home from the set the next morning, I ran to him sobbing like a baby, convinced my life was over. Being the rock that he was, he did his best to assure me I was going to be fine. But the fear raging inside me coupled with the look I saw in his eyes told me a different story.

Two days later I made my way to Beverly Hills to see Dr. K, a noted surgeon and breast specialist. Once seated in his waiting room my eyes caught those of a woman sitting directly across from me in the waiting room. I attempted a half-hearted smile. She politely looked away. Scanning the room for a friendly face, I realized no one was willing to make eye contact. My paranoia tilted to full alert.

After fidgeting in my seat for the longest hour of my life, I was marched into an examination room where I sat alone for another twenty minutes. By the time Dr. K made his entrance, I was beside myself. As I readied to read him the riot act, he reached for my hand, introduced himself, and melted away all my fear and anger. His kind eyes and professional demeanor told me I was in the right place.

Upon completing my exam, he pulled up his rolling stool and looked into my eyes as if he would find the answers to the world in there. It was oddly disconcerting and comforting all at the same time.

"Brenda," he began. "Why did you wait so long to have your breast checked?"

Struggling to hold back tears, I squeaked out the details of my medical journey thus far trying bravely to downplay my fear and failing miserably.

"Did any of your doctors request a needle biopsy?" he inquired.

"No," I said, my whole body heating up in the chill that surrounded me.

He stood, gently touched my shoulder, shook his head, and walked out of the room.

A few minutes later he was back with nurse in tow. "Diane, would you please prepare Mrs. Warner for a biopsy?"

He went on to explain what the procedure entailed and why it was important it be done immediately. As the afternoon light dimmed, my mind swimming with thoughts of more doctors, more hospitals, and more diagnoses, Dr. K performed the biopsy.

"Diane will show you to my office and I'll meet you there when I get the results," he said with a reassuring smile.

Left alone, my sense of dread overtook me. Frantic to find something to take my mind off what was coming, I spotted a bowl of caramels on Dr. K's desk and gobbled them down as if they were the last morsels on earth I would ever eat.

Later, feeling queasy, I searched the room for a blanket or some way of getting warm. I found myself drawn to a corner of the room where a shaft of waning sunlight was streaming in. As I stood there taking in the sun's warmth, I was overcome with a feeling that someone or something else was in the room with me. Glancing around, trying to make sense of what I was feeling, I fell to my knees and prayed.

With tears flowing, so many questions flooded my brain. How did this happen? Was I being punished? Had we made a mistake moving here without the support of friends and family? Was I going to die? My mind offered up one horrible scenario after another as these and more questions exploded in my head.

Illness has a way of bringing you to your knees, forcing you to face your imbalance, notifying you that your body must pay the price for your denial. In this humbled place I realized how precious life is. For the first time I was being confronted with this truth.

In my heart I knew Dr. K would tell me I had breast cancer but no one could have prepared me for the painful reality. Because this lump was sitting directly on my nipple, he was going to have to take my entire breast. Cancer had already claimed my female organs, now it wanted my breast. "God," I thought, "why is this happening to me?"

Dr. K comforted me like a loving father while I fell apart in his arms. When I was able to compose myself, he explained his plan of action. He then called Scott and repeated everything he had told me. He handed me the receiver and left the room.

The only sound on the other end were Scott's muffled sobs. I tried to speak but nothing came out. Finally Scott was able to break the silence.

"Brenda," he said, his voice breaking. "What's the good news?"

"The good news?" I asked, incredulous.

"Us, baby, us. We're the good news."

A strange animal cry involuntarily escaped my body.

"It's us," he went on. "We're together, we're strong and no matter what, we'll be that way through this. We'll do it, Brenda. Together."

At that moment I wanted to time travel into his arms. To feel the physical warmth his words conveyed.

"I love you, Scott," was all I could manage.

"And that's plenty enough for me. I love you too, Bren. Come home. We'll talk about what's next and make a plan."

Dr. K came back into his office and gave me a hug.

"Take your time, Brenda. We're not going anywhere. You do what you have to do. We'll get you through this."

Not wanting the women in the waiting room to know I had been crying, I took a few minutes to fix my face. I stumbled down the hall in a fog and walked into the packed waiting room. Suddenly it hit me, all the reports of breast cancer being on the rise. Here it was in the flesh, a room full of women each waiting to hear her diagnosis.

As I headed out the door I turned one last time to glance at the faces now looking at me. It was in that instant, as I took in the faces of these women, women I didn't know, that I realized we were forever bonded. Forever joined by an experience that would change the trajectory of our lives. We would forever be members of "the club."

6

A Heart and Mind with Separate Lives

I thought getting a diagnosis of cancer was the worst thing that could happen—I was wrong. Accepting my fate and dealing with it on a daily basis was far more difficult. Waking each morning filled with anxiety, I spent my days wondering if I would have a future and at the same time ruminated endlessly about the past. I was obsessed with judgment about everyone and every experience that had led to my current disaster.

Consumed with fear, I experienced firsthand how it drives negative thinking. What I didn't know is where fear comes from. Not an easy question to answer. I believe fear is generated in our unconscious, driven by core beliefs formed in childhood. Those core beliefs, based on the influence of parents, teachers, ministers, and other role models form the basis for our perceptions and consequently our experiences. When we get in touch with the negative beliefs that drive negative thinking, we can begin to heal the underlying patterns that sponsor not only illness and disease, but also fear and separation.

I identified two core beliefs that were responsible for my underlying fear. The first belief, that there was something wrong with me, was forged early in my life. The second belief, that I was not enough, and a closely related sub-belief that I was not capable of handling what came my way, coincided with my first belief. I was eight years old when I experienced a tragedy that, in light of these beliefs, set me on a course that would leave me vulnerable to illness and disease.

It was a hot day. Summer was right around the corner. I boarded the school bus for home, my imagination spinning with plans. I wasn't sure what adventures the summer would hold, but one thing I did know, whatever they were they would include the love of my life, my dog Susie.

I was around three when I started my campaign for a dog. Finally, on my fifth birthday, having worn my parents down, I got Susie. One of our favorite pastimes was climbing into the driver's seat of my parents' old black Oldsmobile and pretending we were traveling the world. I would describe each city we visited in detail while Susie sat at attention, her beautiful brown eyes intently watching every move I made.

Since my father and uncle farmed land together, there were two homes on our property. We occupied one house while my uncle, his wife, their two daughters, and their two dogs lived in the other. Their dogs had a nasty habit of chasing the school bus and biting at the tires so Susie was kept in our fenced backyard, lest she adopt the habit herself.

But on that beautiful almost summer day, someone left the gate open. Susie, on the heels of my cousins' dogs, came running out to greet us. As Susie ran toward the bus, a panicky feeling arose in me. I leaned out the window yelling at her to go home. I heard a yelp as the dual wheels on my side of the bus right where I was sitting went over one of the dogs. I looked out the back window, praying it wasn't Susie.

Suddenly my world turned upside down. There she was, lying in the middle of the road. As fear and pain shot through me I bolted from my seat toward the front of the bus screaming, "NO! NO! NO!"

Bursting through the door I ran to her, hoping with all my heart she was still alive. Seeing her motionless form I quickly realized she was already gone.

I pulled her broken body into my arms, sobbing, *"Please God, please! I'll be good . . . I'll behave . . . I promise! Please God, bring Susie back*!"

But it was not to be. My beloved Susie had been taken from me. Was this my punishment from God for being a bad person?

Believing there is something wrong with you often translates into believing you are a bad person. You draw into your life the circumstances and experiences that mirror those beliefs. Without the understanding that all our experiences, good or bad, are here to help us grow into more loving, compassionate, expanded beings, we suffer.

I was too young to understand this experience wasn't meant to make me suffer. Nor did I have parents that understood this concept. As a result, negative beliefs were fortified instead of healed. They passed down from generation to generation resulting in a life in which I felt victimized by a fearful punishing God and a cruel unfair world.

I can't speak directly to what my parents experienced but I can say they had no idea how to deal with my pain. They did their best to distract me trying to establish a new normal. For me, normal no longer existed. I was in pain. More pain than I had ever felt before and no distraction big or small was going to make things normal again.

With my parents unable to help me feel better, I withdrew. I now had proof that love equaled pain. That God couldn't be trusted and there was no one to love or care for me. I was now on my own in a hard cruel world.

Saying no to love became my protection as this pattern began to overshadow everything in my life. I moved away from the sensitive young girl with a big heart and took on the role of "angry loner," determined to prove to God and everyone else she didn't need them.

Making this decision only served to cement my erroneous belief that there was something wrong with me. And to further serve my pain, I began having experiences that proved my theory. As my anger turned into resentment, I became more and more convinced that life was unfair and not worth living.

Sensing my withdrawal, my parents became desperate to get me back on track and insisted I finish the school year as a way to help me move on. But their decision backfired when my teacher sent me home because I was despondent. Growing weary of my attitude, they tried to convince me that while Susie's death was tragic, there were other dogs out there that needed good homes. "After all," my father commented one night at dinner, "Susie was just a dog, and dogs can be replaced!"

Losing Susie was extremely painful, but what added to my pain was pretending to be someone I wasn't, closing myself off to love. In full protective mode, I pushed away anyone or anything that tried to ease my burden. The lonely, angry, resentful me was determined to punish God and anyone else who got too close, stressing my system, making it possible for my dis-ease to become my disease.

Being that there is an undeniable emotional component to illness, it is no coincidence that in the weeks and months that followed Susie's death I was diagnosed with ulcerative colitis, among a host of other physical ailments. Unresolved, unexpressed emotions create havoc and over time stress the body. To protect ourselves we take on roles instead of living our true nature. We close our hearts because we equate love with pain. Rather than really living we are merely coping, playing roles that are often opposite of who we are.

In James Van Praagh's book *Unfinished Business*, he says fear is a normal emotional response that is part of our survival instinct. But fear directed toward anything other than survival is pure illusion. Fear that there's something wrong with us, that we're not enough, that we're not worthy of love, or that we lack anything are not beliefs steeped in truth. But this illusory belief system is the very place dis-ease begins when we are unable to heal the false perceptions that drive unhealthy patterns and behaviors.

I spent a lifetime blaming others for my lot in life. It's a lot easier to blame outside circumstances for why life isn't working than to take responsibility for our choices. When blame becomes a way of life, this pattern establishes the belief that we are victims with no control over our lives. But that is only part of the story. While we may not have control over circumstances in our lives, my losing Susie for example, we do have a choice as to how we respond to those circumstances. This can be a bitter pill to swallow but living in denial of this truth keeps us stuck in a perpetual cycle of blame and victimization, leading to further problems.

Each day we witness the consequences of living unconsciously. We deny the power of love, turning over control to our egos without realizing we have a choice. We can choose to examine the thoughts and beliefs that leave us feeling powerless, doing whatever is necessary to heal or we can choose to live as victims, believing the world is out to get us. Being accountable, taking responsibility for our feelings and actions heals not only our bodies but also holds the key to healing the whole of society.

When we deny our feelings, shutting love out of our lives, we invite trouble. Left unattended, what is repressed and denied in us will eventually surface, begging us to pay attention so we can heal. Faced with cancer yet again I was getting this lesson in ever-increasing doses. And just to prove I was stronger than any cancer, my resistance leapt into action to defeat this enemy.

What I didn't know is that in resistance I was powerless to make any real change or invite healing. But this time the cancer was sending me a very strong message that said it was no longer acceptable for me to live my life the way I had been living it. My options? Change or die!

Resistance is a form of fear that comes up when we make the decision to confront our demons. Early on we are conditioned to believe what resistance tells us—that we don't have what it takes to move through our problems and heal our lives. In the case of illness and disease, our conditioning informs us that they are strictly a physical problem. This not only excuses us from taking responsibility for our emotional and spiritual healing, but also demands we look outside ourselves for the answer. Being told we are genetically pre-disposed to a certain disease only adds fuel to this fire. However, pre-disposed or not, we are responsible for healing the underlying causes of disease.

It has been scientifically proven that genes can be turned on and off. In Dr. Bruce Lipton's book *Biology of Belief*, he explains the science behind the fact that we can and do have a positive effect on illness and disease when we willingly and courageously face our problems. When we are willing to heal the negative thinking, behaviors, and beliefs that sponsor ill health, when we acknowledge that the physical body is connected to the whole of us—mind, body, and spirit—and must be involved in the healing process, we can begin to heal.

And I do mean heal, not cure. A cure generally involves surgery and/or prescription medications. While there is certainly nothing wrong with taking these steps, they generally deal with symptoms only, not the underlying cause of illness and disease. All illness and disease begins in the spiritual body where dis-ease interrupts the flow of energy. Jim Self, a wonderful teacher/healer and recurring guest host on our radio show, Conscious Talk Radio, describes this beautifully. He says, when we are young, going along our merry way, our natural state is ease. Then, along comes a parent or someone we look up to who says something mean-spirited, like how stupid or ugly we are, and because of their undue influence, we adopt this as our truth.

Once this happens, ease is immediately turned into dis-ease. This dis-ease creates negative feelings that become part of the emotional body and over time the impact of the dis-ease erodes the self, opening up the opportunity for disease and illness to manifest in the physical.

When we focus on a cure, we fight disease on the physical level only, missing the actual root cause. A healthier more natural way of approaching this is to use our energy to focus on wellness and ways to work with the body. At the same time we must also take steps to address the negative patterns and beliefs that sponsored the illness in the first place. This healing approach creates an environment for the body to re-balance and harmonize, and given the opportunity, it will.

Once we embrace our healing, moving forward both emotionally and spiritually, we still have the options of medication and/or a procedure. But until we get to the bottom of what's causing the problem, we risk having that problem or something similar show up again. And when that happens, it can sometimes come back with a vengeance.

True healing brings up tremendous fear because it requires us to make the commitment to change. Diseases are fed and nurtured by our lifestyles: what we eat, think, believe, how well we care for ourselves, our stress levels, how loving our relationships are, and many other personal choices. The work that is required to bring balance so the body has the opportunity to heal can be daunting. By contrast, taking a pill or submitting to a procedure doesn't require self-examination or a change in lifestyle.

But making the choice to heal, though scary, can open up life in ways we never could have imagined. One of the most powerful is the opportunity to forgive ourselves our perceived shortcomings and mistakes. This in turn allows us to reach out and forgive those we feel have wronged us. Acknowledging this divine part of our humanity can create an environment that is very conducive to healing.

Through forgiveness, compassion is awakened and creates an internal shift that will guide you through your healing process. As you continue this process your heart opens allowing feelings of gratitude, maybe for the first time in years. Feeling gratitude for yourself, your circumstances, and all of life contains potent healing energy that grows exponentially each time you expand your capacity to give and receive love.

However, this is easier said than done. Particularly when the mind convinces you you're not capable of succeeding on this path, as mine did. Even deeper in my soul I knew if I didn't move in this direction I might not live. I stuck with it because for the first time, I was determined to change my life and heal the parts of me that were broken.

I tell you this because it's natural to fall back into old patterns of thinking and reacting in times of great challenge. It's also natural to feel confused and fearful when you start something new. Let yourself off the hook by allowing yourself to be with your confusion and fear without trying to escape your feelings. I found that when I allowed myself to breathe into the fear and confusion, those feelings dissipated. And when I practiced this religiously, I felt calm and empowered to continue on.

When it comes to matters of God and the heart, the mind doesn't know how to integrate these energies. The mind is good at analyzing, interpreting and conjuring up past experiences and future fears. But when it comes to problem-solving, the mind cannot access our innate wisdom, particularly at the level of healing that is required when dealing with disease.

The shift from mind to heart where our connection to God is present doesn't happen overnight. This is a transformational process requiring patience and a deep desire to surrender everything you think you know. One of the best ways to connect with Spirit is to breathe into your heart until you feel at peace. Then, request that your heart make its wisdom known while at the same time being aware. That is when your mind will likely begin its chatter, which is normal; don't fight it. Instead, be willing to let your thoughts come and go as you refocus on your breathing and your intention to connect. Remember, the mind is used to being in control so a retraining period is natural.

Because I was in the infancy stages of learning about this and still at the mercy of my mind, there were endless dark days when I was filled with doubt. My mind worked desperately to convince me I wasn't capable of healing. When my energy was low I bought into the chatter, spiraling down, listening to my mind tell me over and over that I needed professional help. Of course, this was not possible. Our financial picture was dismal. We paid our bills but at the end of every month we were lucky to have twenty or thirty dollars in our collective pocket. Paying for therapy was not an option, particularly since we didn't have insurance. My fear, driven by shame, wouldn't allow me to ask my parents or Scott's for help so I continued to confront my negative self-talk head on, breathing through the strong emotions of fear that accompanied my thoughts.

The mind is masterful at offering up its interpretation of a solution and then creating another problem that needs to be solved before we even have time to think about solving the initial problem. The mind cannot solve our problems. It can only keep us in a perpetual state of confusion, drama, and fear while offering up one useless theory after another. Meanwhile, our lives continue to fall apart.

If you are facing your own demons, you may be operating on some of the very same beliefs that ran my life. Beliefs like, you don't know how to access what you need, you can't have what you desire, life is hard, you never get what you want, or you're not capable, lovable, or worthy. Please be persistent. Have faith that you're more than capable. God hears our prayers, God knows our heart's desires and God loves us beyond measure. We are part of the God presence, expressing in human form. In other words, we are spiritual beings having a human experience and as this God presence, possessing the power to transform our lives.

In the early stages of assembling my spiritual toolbox with new concepts, ideas, rituals, and breathing techniques to support me on my healing journey, I discovered meditation. In my first attempt, I took a candle into my small walk-in closet hoping the flame would help me concentrate enough to put me in a meditative state. That was a mistake! Not only did I almost burn my apartment down, the smoke from the candle almost suffocated me. Needless to say, I was thrilled to find that simply by breathing into my body I was able to get beyond my mind and connect with God in meditation.

In the beginning, I fully expected to reach a place where peace already existed in me but that was an unreal expectation. Reaching nirvana every time you meditate, particularly when you're just learning, is unrealistic. This is why staying committed to the process and releasing expectations are so important. Without that vigilance you will be tempted to throw up your arms and walk away giving the mind exactly what it wants, to remain in control.

I remember one day in particular when I was having trouble quieting my mind. In the middle of my breathing process two thoughts began to surface over and over despite my attempts to ignore them. First, how would Scott handle having a wife with only one breast? And the other, how was I going to cope with losing a breast and its devastating effect on my self-image? Instead of following my own advice and allowing these thoughts to flow through, my mind hooked in and fear took over.

Once fear had me in its grip, other fearful thoughts began to surface. I found myself reminiscing about the time my father and I were playing ball together in our backyard. As we took turns throwing to each other, Dad talked about wanting nine boys to form his own baseball team. As I listened, I began to feel guilty about being born a girl and consequently began the denial of my femininity.

Now, having lost my female organs to cervical cancer and faced with the loss of my breast, I knew I needed to break that pattern. I needed to start appreciating my feminine body and myself as a woman. I started taking candlelight baths twice a day while I listened to music that moved and inspired me. In the evenings, instead of watching television, I enjoyed quiet time reading self-help books. During the day I scheduled leisurely walks in nature devoting time to appreciate my life.

Granted, these were small steps. I had a long way to go to reclaim myself and restore my health. But doing these few simple things was an important milestone for me in my march toward wellness. I was sending a clear message to the Universe. I was ready, willing, and able to honor life, to honor myself and to take responsibility for my part in all of it. If only it were that easy.

7

Confronting Reality

As my surgery consultation with Dr. K was fast approaching, I realized taking care of myself was vital to a successful operation and recovery. It was also essential to my relationship with Scott. He loved the tender side of me that I found so difficult to expose. But with some of the newfound lessons I was learning and applying, he was beginning to see and feel the difference.

Scott and I discussed in detail the questions we had for Dr. K. First and foremost we wanted to know my chances of survival and if there were any alternatives besides taking my breast. Though he had already told me saving my breast was impossible, I wanted to make sure he had investigated all options before making his final decision.

"Brenda," Dr. K said, reaching for my hands. "I'm afraid there's no way we can save your breast. As I explained before, we won't know anything for sure until after your surgery is complete. There are many variables to consider, such as the type of cancer you have, whether it's localized or not, and whether there are any infected lymph nodes. Your chances right now for survival are good, but it's best you stay positive and focus your energy on surgery, not on trying to save your breast." With that he squeezed my hands and waited for my response.

As I struggled to speak, Scott interceded. Immediately my mind started the chatter. How much was this going to cost? How much of a burden was it going be on Scott? How much work was this going to be for everyone? I was reminded that after surgery there would be treatment. And if my past held any clue to my future, things weren't going to work out very well for me. Death, my mind informed me, might be my only way out.

In the midst of this surreal discussion I desperately tried to find my center to breathe into my heart and find some peace. It was hopeless—my mind was in control. Fear had found its place and focused breathing was impossible. With every negative thought that flashed through my mind, I sank deeper and deeper into fear; further and further away from my center as Scott and Dr. K continued their conversation.

Struggling to stay focused on what was happening, I suddenly heard Dr. K tell Scott we needed to give the hospital a down payment before he could admit me. Slam! I was back in the conversation.

"Consequently, Scott, I can't stress how important it is that the money be paid right away. We want to make sure Brenda has every advantage to heal. I don't want her to be put at risk of not making a full recovery because all of the funds are not in place."

"That's not a problem, Dr. K," I heard Scott say. "We'll have the money in a couple of days."

Not a problem? I thought. *Not a problem? What is he talking about? A couple of days? We don't have two nickels to rub together. Where were we going to get this kind of money?*

On the way home, I pushed Scott for answers.

"Why did you promise Dr. K we'd have the money in a couple days? Why didn't you ask if there were any other options?"

"Don't worry about it, Brenda. I'll take care of it," he replied calmly.

"You'll take care of it?" I said, my voice reaching levels out of my control. "How are you going to 'take care of it'?"

"Calm down, Brenda."

"Don't tell me to calm down! Why would you make a promise you know we can't keep?"

Of course, he didn't have the answers. But I kept at him, goading us into a full-scale argument.

By the time we walked through our apartment door we were both furious. Exhaustion overwhelmed me. To avoid further confrontation, I jumped into bed and pulled the covers over my head. I prayed that by morning there would be a solution, knowing there wouldn't. I fell into a fitful sleep.

Later that night before going to work, Scott woke me wanting to apologize but I let him have it again. As he stomped out of the room, I turned over and tried to get back to sleep. As I drifted off, I heard a voice. It told me to trust, all would be well. *Uh huh*, I thought. *That's easy for you to say.*

The following morning, as I crawled out of bed feeling like a truck had run over me, the phone rang. A friend from Seattle was on the other end saying he was coming to Los Angeles on business and wanted to come by for a visit. And though it seemed the last thing we needed, Scott and I agreed that some company might be a good diversion.

His visit turned out to be nothing short of a miracle. He not only opened his heart to our problem but also offered to pay the up-front costs of my surgery. Were my prayers really being answered? I was beginning to think it might be a good idea to trust this voice I was hearing.

With the burden of funding settled, it was time to inform family and friends. We called Scott's parents first and as expected they were kind and supportive. There was no discussion about finances or if we needed any help. Scott already owed them money and though it was clear they loved and supported us, it was also clear it wasn't going to express itself in a financial way.

After speaking with our friends, the last call we made was to my parents. Relieved that my father wasn't home, I spoke with my mother who assured me my father would insist on coming to LA for my surgery. That was the last thing I needed.

"It's really not necessary for you to come, Mom. I mean I appreciate the gesture but it's minor surgery. I'll be out of the hospital the same day so really there wouldn't be anything for you to do."

I hated lying to her but I justified it because I didn't want to hurt her or God forbid, cause another argument. I knew I was looking at at least two, maybe three days in the hospital and depending on if the cancer had spread, maybe more. But I couldn't face the prospect of taking care of them when I really needed to be taking care of me.

She didn't buy the story about my surgery being minor and continued to press me. As I struggled to answer her questions, my father walked in and my mother abruptly handed him the phone. After hearing me out, he reacted as if nothing I said mattered. They were coming to LA and that was that!

I felt the heat of anger rise in me. Why did he never listen to me or give credence to my desires? I wanted to lash out at him for being such a jerk. Instead, I swallowed my feelings and kept quiet. After hanging up I turned to Scott for moral support, only to find he was on my father's side. He thought I would regret not allowing my parents to participate and the last thing I needed right now was to feel regret. As hard as it was to hear this, I had to admit he was right.

That night, as I struggled with my feelings of guilt, I made one last attempt to breathe into my body and open my heart. I prayed for guidance. Within moments, I heard something I wasn't prepared to hear: *All that matters is love.*

As the days quickly passed leading to my parents' arrival, my anxiety increased. Every day I practiced my breathing, and every day I struggled to stay centered. Had I known that by focusing on what I didn't want I was actually drawing those experiences to me, I would have done things differently. I didn't yet understand how our life experience reflects our thinking. I was unaware of how the past plays into this scenario. I didn't understand that ruminating about the past, about what I didn't want, would bring more of the same.

This pattern is activated by the strong emotions that come into play when we feel we're not getting what we want. Being smack-dab in the middle of a life-threatening disease can present all manner of life-changing opportunities. But that can only happen if we have an awareness of this potential and open our eyes and hearts to a better way. If not, we miss the precious lesson being offered and continue to repeat old patterns.

When my parents arrived, I was surprised I was glad to see them. However, my good feelings didn't last. Small talk had always been the way we interacted, but this time was different. This time I was craving connection. This time I was hoping we could have a real conversation. That didn't happen. True to form our conversations focused on the trivial: LA traffic, LA life and other equally innocuous subjects. Anything to avoid discussing what was really going on.

I found myself going on automatic. I realized my parents weren't going to broach the subject of my cancer or what the future held. And, true to form, I was too scared to bring it up myself. I began withdrawing into my own little world where I would try to find a way to engage my parents, to tell them how I was feeling.

My father, being an avid smoker, had to have his cigarettes. He knew how I felt about his smoking but he didn't care. Not only was I furious about him killing himself, but his utter disregard of me in light of my condition enraged me. As usual, I couldn't bring myself to say anything, and as usual, I stuffed my anger and politely suggested he smoke on the lanai.

Mom started in as soon as he left the room. She ranted about his "nasty habit" until she had worked herself into a frenzy. Observing her, I had a realization: she used my father's smoking as a trigger to release her emotions instead of admitting what she was really feeling. I realized also that as a family we had fine-tuned this method to legendary proportions and I held the prize for swallowing my feelings, having learned how much safer that was than telling my truth. Also accepting that taking care of another's needs was far more important than tending to my own, I found myself consoling my mother instead of dealing with what was going on.

Later, as I was putting away the last of their belongings I tried to envision my future. And while my spirit was trying to hold a vision of life, my mind was filled with persistent thoughts of dying. Somewhere in the middle of this fear fest I heard the voice say, *It isn't time for you to leave yet.* But before I could really latch on to it, my mother interrupted me telling me my father was lighting up, again.

The familiarity of this scene struck me like a bolt of lightning. Throughout childhood my parents and their problems had always trumped what was going on in my life, and in my marriage to Bob I unwittingly continued that dynamic. It was as if I was invisible. Unless of course, I was ill. When I was ill I got all the attention I needed from all three of them.

I began to wonder if there was a part of me that was using my illnesses to get what I wanted and needed from the people I loved. If this was true, and I wanted to survive, it was imperative for me to heal what was driving this pattern of behavior.

Throughout my journey, I have been reminded over and over that profound awareness comes to us when we are ready for our lives to be different. But for the new to be birthed into consciousness and practically applied in our lives, we must embrace the truth of our unconscious behavior. If we are to transcend what is threatening our wellbeing, we must be willing to accept that change is our only option. This requires courage and patience. For me, exploring how I could change these long-held patterns was a challenge. My mind was relentless in its attempts to convince me that I didn't know how to live a different life.

The conscious mind is masterful at filling our heads with stories of negativity and failure. I've learned the hard way that the desire to have our lives be different won't happen until we're truly ready to surrender the patterns that keep us from the life we want. Once resistance is transformed into surrender, magic happens.

Of course, I was far from being able to surrender and take responsibility for my life, but for the first time, there was a glimmer of hope. Little by little I was waking up, realizing things I had never thought about before, much less desired to change. And with each new concept my desire to move beyond my negative thinking and patterns was strengthening.

In the midst of all this, Scott was working grueling hours to pay bills and put food on our table. Looking back, his absence was a plus as he and my father were prone to butting heads. While Scott was not the kind of person to look for trouble, he was very protective of me, especially when it came to the dynamic with my father.

In a conversation, my dad expressed his surprise at how much time Scott was gone at work. I told him he had a demanding job that required long hours. And though this wasn't the whole truth, we were desperate for money, which forced Scott to work a grueling schedule. I purposely kept this from my parents, not needing to be reminded that my father had been right about us quitting our good-paying jobs in Seattle to run off to LA in search of some "pipe dream." Yes, maybe we had been foolish. But foolish or not this was our life and we felt we were entitled to make our own mistakes.

The only bright spot in the days leading up to my surgery came when I received a phone call from my close friend Carlene. We had met when I was living in Seattle and had instantly become friends. When I told her about my condition she jumped to my support saying she wanted to be by my side. Yes, it would mean another person in our cramped apartment but the support I knew she would provide trumped inconvenience.

Upon her arrival she worked her magic diffusing the tension that surrounded us with laughter and light. The anxiety in my family was an all too familiar state of being. The mood in my childhood home was always serious. Carlene had the ability to look at life through the lens of laughter and go with the flow, something I admired in her and desired for myself but had been unable to achieve.

Even with Carlene's influence I struggled with the bad feelings between my father and me. And though it was my deep desire to have some healing between us before my surgery, I couldn't let go of the notion that he should make the first move. After all, he had caused the pain between us in the first place. He should be the one to apologize for his behavior.

In retrospect I know it was silly to hold out but at the time I was too stubborn to admit my shortcomings and be the bigger person. I wasn't aware my taking this stance was hurting me far worse than it was hurting him. In many ways I was no different from my dad when it came to my need to be right. This similarity between us only added to why it was almost impossible for us to connect.

With surgery drawing near and Scott working so many hours, he and I desperately needed time alone. His absence and our mounting debt were taking a toll on our relationship. I wanted to share what was in my heart. I wanted him to know how much I loved him and that I couldn't bear to think of my life without him. With no privacy to carve out the time and space to talk, I tucked my feelings away, praying that after surgery when everyone was gone, we'd each be able to share what was in our hearts.

Walking through the hospital doors on the day of surgery, my pulse was racing. In a few short hours, my future would unfold before me. That thought alone was terrifying. Once settled in my room, thoughts of my father drifted through my mind. I knew I had to pray— pray for help in letting go of my past, help in releasing my negative thoughts and feelings, help in opening my heart to love. My deepest desire was to awaken from surgery and feel that love. Then, and only then would I be able to tell my father he was forgiven and open the space for us to begin anew.

8

Divine Intervention

Before I knew it, I was back in my room, a nurse injecting something into my IV bag. The room started to spin as queasiness overtook me. Moments later, through my haze, I heard her tell someone, "Don't worry. It's common for patients to have reactions to certain anesthetics." Though still in a fog, I was coherent enough to know this wasn't my issue. In recovery I had regained consciousness a few times and wasn't nauseous at all. It was only after I was injected with this unknown medication that I felt sick.

As I drifted in and out of consciousness, I became aware that someone was standing by my bed trying to get my attention. It was my friend Carly, not to be confused with Carlene, from New York. We had spoken recently but I didn't know she was going to be in LA during my surgery. I had met Carly, who was a trained hypnotherapist, at a seminar a few years earlier. Her appearance at my bedside felt heaven-sent as she began to work her magic on me.

In spite of my state I responded to her hypnotic suggestions and was under within moments. A half hour later I was sitting up, asking for something to eat. My parents, Carlene and my friend Eric, also there to support me, were so impressed that they asked her to do a group session to ease their anxiety. Though she was hesitant about accomplishing what they wanted, she agreed, joking with my father that she was going to use them as her guinea pigs.

As I lay there, watching the transformation of the group's frantic state, I couldn't help but note that Carly had miraculously appeared when I needed her. As I added up the "coincidences;" Art arriving at the precise moment we needed financial help; Carlene and Eric, both angels that loved and supported me; and now Carly, I was beginning to believe that there *was* someone or something watching over me.

In the short time we'd lived in LA, Scott and I had met a wonderful group of friends. The day following my surgery many of them stopped by. Before long my room was filled with laughter, love, and flowers. Everyone was having a great time. Everyone that is, except my mother. As the day wore on she became more and more distant, sitting in the corner by the window, in a world of her own.

Later that day after our friends had gone home, Mom continued her vigil in the corner while Dad, Eric, Carlene and Scott decided to go get something to eat. Mom declined saying she wanted to keep an eye on me. As the room emptied and quiet invaded the space, I realized how exhausted I was. Distracted by what was bothering Mom I couldn't rest until I found out.

"Mom?"

"Hmm?"

"Are you okay?" I ventured.

"I am so disappointed in you, Brenda." she exploded. "How could you have paid more attention to your friends than to your father and me? We drove a thousand miles to be here and you don't seem to appreciate that at all."

Hurt and taken aback, I felt defensive. I wanted to tell her it was because my friends had very busy lives and it was my only chance to be with them. My parents, on the other hand, were staying while I convalesced and there would be plenty of alone time. This is what I wanted to share with her, but instead, not wanting to add fuel to the fire, I kept my mouth shut.

History had taught me this was the safest way through these minefields, so I apologized for making her feel uncomfortable. I apologized because I felt guilty. I apologized because I was the one who had put everyone in this position.

Accepting my apology she dried her eyes, hugged me and went off to eat while I was left to deal with the emotional fallout. As I lay there going over what she said, a memory of another display of her jealousy surfaced.

One day I called to tell her that my then boyfriend was taking me to Hawaii, all expenses paid.

"It must be nice to have someone foot the bill for a week in Hawaii," she retorted.

I was so shocked by her tone that I didn't know how to respond. I had expected she would be excited for me, but her snarky response hurt me deeply, and as had become my pattern, I buried my feelings, vowing to keep my mouth shut about what was happening in my life. But now, with so many parts of my life illuminated by my cancer, I somehow knew I was going to be forced to deal with my feelings. Stuffing them inside, pretending things were right with me when they weren't, was about to be blown apart. It was time to tell Mom my truth. But how could I do it without exploding? So much anger, sadness, guilt, and resentment had built walls around my heart. I knew that until I could come to terms with my own feelings, talking to her would only create more problems.

Disappointment and an acute awareness of the mess I had perpetuated overwhelmed me. Filled with anxiety, I tried to get comfortable. That's when I noticed my breast was hurting. Why now, I wondered? I had been pain-free most of the day. At that moment something clicked. Could there be a connection between what just happened with my mom and the pain in my breast? What if my breast was the receptacle of all the negative feelings I had stuffed inside over the years? And what if my body had finally reached its zenith and was crying out?

On the heels of these thoughts the pain in my breast intensified. Shifting my position to try and get comfortable, I heard, "Breathe." I resisted. But my resistance only made the pain worse. I finally acquiesced, breathing into my body, as the tears stinging my cheeks turned into gigantic sobs.

After a good long cry, the pain in my breast began to ease. The pain in my heart did not. One good cry wasn't going to change a lifetime of disappointment and overwhelming feelings of inadequacy. Nor was it going to change the fact that suppressing all my negative feelings over the years might be one of the reasons I was now laying in this hospital bed with cancer.

As these thoughts rambled through my mind, I thought about how grateful I was to have the support of wonderful friends like Eric and Carly. When I first met Eric, several months before my illness was diagnosed, we bumped into each other like two old friends meeting up again after a long vacation apart. Eric and Scott felt that same intense bond too, and Eric quickly became an integral part of our lives.

After my surgery, he was there for me in every way. He took time off work to help out and assisted my parents any way he could. He was a Christian with a strong faith in God and always walked the talk. He also had a great sense of humor and tremendous compassion. We talked a lot about God and what it meant to have faith. We also laughed a lot, which was something I treasured.

Eric was always looking out for the other guy. That morning in my hospital room as Carly was hypnotizing everyone, the phone next to me began to ring. Eric, hoping to stop the noise from disturbing everyone, lunged to grab it and everyone was able to maintain the altered state. Eric was not so lucky since he was jolted out of his hypnotic trance.

Later he complained he wasn't feeling well. He said he felt like he wasn't attached to his body. I subsequently learned that sometimes happens when one is in an altered state and suddenly snapped back to consciousness by a disturbing noise or quick movement. After telling me how he was feeling, I called Carly to ask if something could be done. She understood immediately and said she would be happy to come back that evening and help him back into his body.

Eric arrived first and clearly wasn't himself. Once Carly got there, Eric explained, "I feel like I've been dragging an extra body around all day."

She assured him once she hypnotized him and brought him out properly, he'd be fine.

"Let's take advantage of the empty bed here. I want you to lie down and begin breathing mindfully," she instructed.

As Eric settled in, Carly went to work.

"Is there something you want to talk about? Anything that's bothering you?" she inquired.

He hesitated, mumbling something about his concern for my recovery. It was like Eric to worry about me but I knew there was something far more important for him to explore.

Early on Eric and I had bonded over family values and those myriad of challenges we all have with parents and siblings. He talked about many issues he had with his father that weren't resolved before his death. Armed with this information, I encouraged Carly to explore it.

"Eric, tell me about the last time you were with your father," Carly directed softly.

"It was the day he was scheduled for heart surgery," he said without hesitation.

This information gave Carly a place to start the conversation. She suggested Eric go back to that day and talk to his father. Within moments he was describing the scene. He was standing at the foot of his father's bed.

Ever the humorist, he said, "He was connected to a plethora of life-support equipment and tubing that looked like a plumber's nightmare."

Carly smiled and suggested he share his thoughts about the problems between them. What happened next took us both by surprise. The look on Eric's face changed. It was clear he was in conversation with his father. He confronted him about leaving his mother to live with their next-door neighbor. After a few moments, Carly asked that Eric allow his father to speak through him in response to what was being said. But before Carly could get the last word out, Eric curled up in a ball and began to sob as he described the pain his father was feeling for betraying his family.

When the crying stopped, Eric said, "I want to forgive my father."

Carly encouraged him to do so. Feeling the silence had gone on too long, she asked, "What's happening, Eric?"

He described where he and his father were. "It's completely dark except for hundreds of wandering souls floating around, souls that look like illuminated jellyfish."

Astonished at the scene Eric was describing, Carly asked him to continue.

After a brief moment he explained, "In order to go from one place to another you merely 'will' yourself to move. You don't need to physically walk or talk."

Carly knew this was the perfect time to bring Eric back to full consciousness and was about to do so when suddenly Eric's face contorted and he cried out, "No . . . there's a beast! A beast is stalking us!"

Carly quickly commanded, "Eric, take a deep breath and when you're ready, look the beast directly in its eyes and tell it to go away."

Eric took a breath and said, "In the name of the flesh and blood of Jesus Christ my Lord, I command you to leave me now!"

For several moments there was silence as we both waited anxiously. Finally, Eric reported that on his command the beast had vanished. When Carly asked him to describe what this beast looked like he said, "It has the body of a human and the head of an insect."

As Carly and I digested this information we noticed Eric's breathing had slowed considerably.

Soon, unprompted by Carly he said, "I'm being drawn toward a bright light."

Carly reached for Eric's wrist and felt his pulse.

"Eric," she said, "Listen to me. Let your father go into the light. Let him go, Eric. You come here, to this time and place."

But he resisted, mumbling something about going home.

Carly began to panic, telling me if she wasn't able to convince Eric to let his father go on without him, we could lose him.

Without thinking I bolted out of bed and grabbed Eric's hand, "Eric!" I pleaded. "Please come back. Eric, please! I need you. Scott needs you. Please, Eric, don't leave us now. Please!"

Despite my efforts he continued to pull away. I was about to get a nurse when Eric began to speak. He was barely audible. Listening closely, we were able to make out that he and his father were floating in the middle of thousands of souls that were hovering above Jesus as he hung on the cross.

Mesmerized by what he was telling us, Carly tried once more to bring him back. Eric began to weep.

"Eric," she asked quietly, "why are you crying?"

"Jesus," he sobbed. "I'm watching Jesus look toward the heavens. He's waiting. Waiting to give up his earthly body."

Just then at the foot of Eric's bed, something caught my eye. For one brief moment I thought I saw the silhouette of Christ. I blinked a couple of times in disbelief to clear my senses. When I looked again the silhouette of Christ was still there.

Eric broke my spell as he began telling us that he, along with all the other souls around him, were stroking the face of Jesus, trying to absorb his pain. Just then his body began to shake uncontrollably. At that point Carly grabbed Eric's shoulders. She motioned for me to grab his feet to keep him on the bed. Moments later Eric took a long deep breath while stretching his arms to his side as if he were hanging on a cross. He stayed in that position for several minutes. Suddenly his body went limp and his breathing came back to normal. Carly was finally able to gain control and within minutes had Eric back to full consciousness. Wonder and relief washing over me, I knelt at his side and silently gave a prayer of thanks.

When Eric felt steady enough to move he slowly made his way to the chair next to me and sat, without saying a word. Carly took her place in the chair on the other side of my bed. Without a word we reached for each other's hands. Sitting in silence, aware that something extraordinary had taken place, not one of us had the words to express what we were feeling.

Several minutes passed before I was finally able to offer a prayer of gratitude. Without saying a word, Carly and Eric left. I snuggled in and for the first time in months, fell into a deep, peaceful sleep.

9

Emotional Rollercoaster

The next morning I awoke embraced by a wonderful sense of peace. After breakfast I reached out to Eric and Carly to talk about what had happened the night before. Besides telling Scott, we decided it would be best to keep it to ourselves. We knew how an event like this could be misunderstood or even dismissed completely and we didn't want to give anyone the opportunity to discredit the profound experience we had shared.

Though I hadn't had the direct encounter Eric had, the light and shadow phenomena of Christ was real for me. Somehow knowing this gave me a renewed sense of inner strength and resolve that I hadn't had prior to my surgery. Eric reached a new level of acceptance with his father and Carly felt blessed to have been the catalyst. It had been a transcendent experience none of us would forget.

Scheduled to be released later that day I was eager for Dr. K's post-op consultation. When he arrived he got right down to business.

"We removed fifteen lymph nodes that are on their way to the lab for testing. I'm concerned that because the tumor was in your breast for almost two years that it has quite probably infected your lymph. I feel strongly we should explore the possibility of chemotherapy."

A stunned silence filled the room as I tried to make sense of what he had said. "Why would I want to make myself sicker while at the same time trying to be well?" I asked him.

As my hands involuntarily formed into fists and my third chakra tightened, I wondered if my reaction was merely classic fear. Who would choose to go down this road if given any other option? Who would volunteer for hair loss, bouts of nausea, and no guarantee the cancer wouldn't return in spite of treatment? Who would willingly sign up for treatments that had been proven to cause a whole rash of other health issues?

To calm me, Dr. K reluctantly agreed to wait for my biopsy results before proceeding. Although relieved at his acquiescence, I knew this would not be the last I would hear on the matter. But every time the subject of chemotherapy came up, my body reacted the same way. With this repeated response pattern it became more and more evident these reactions were a signal to move in another direction. Which direction, I had no idea, but the feeling was too strong to ignore.

Explaining this to family and friends was futile since they dismissed my reactions as a response to high anxiety. Throughout my illness I had repeatedly pushed aside my intuition, blindly obeying doctors' orders. This time I was determined that things would be different. This time I was going to follow my inner guidance and give my body what it wanted. I was also determined not to listen to friends and family simply because I was feeling insecure and they thought they knew better. Something inside me was changing, urging me to make my own decisions. I wasn't sure what was driving this change but I felt it had something to do with the experience in my hospital room. Regardless of the reason, this was the first time since my ordeal began that I felt clearly guided to take charge of my own recovery.

My hospital stay had been an emotional rollercoaster but nothing could deter me from clinging to the amazing events of the night before. I was committed to moving through the rest of the experience with a positive attitude. However, my resolve was short-lived. As a rollercoaster travels, what goes up must come down. My down came that morning after I was released.

With Scott still working nights and sleeping during the day, it fell on my parents to take me home. As we made our way through the parking garage looking for our car, Dad announced they were going to stay another week. They felt with Carly headed back to New York, Carlene headed home and Eric going back to work, I would need them.

I had mixed feelings about their plan. On the one hand, I appreciated the gesture, while on the other I knew their staying was sure to bring trouble, especially with my father. I didn't know when but I knew that sooner or later it was inevitable. I could feel his "I told you so" lecture lurking in the wings.

Unaware at the time that we get what we expect, I didn't fully appreciate the dynamic I had set in play. I was expecting trouble and trouble was poised to accommodate. As we approached the car, my father started complaining about driving in LA traffic.

Continuing his rant he abruptly turned to me and said, "It looks like you're in pretty good shape so driving won't be a problem," and threw the keys to me.

Stunned stupid by his request, I agreed. I had learned long ago that accommodating my father was the smart thing to do if I wanted to avoid an argument. But before I could get into the driver's seat, my mother interceded.

"What are you thinking?" she started. "Brenda has just been through an incredible ordeal and is in no shape to be driving, particularly in this insane place!" She continued speaking of me as if I weren't there. "Let me remind you we came here for Brenda. Maybe just this once you could think of someone beside yourself!"

My father, never one to be questioned in the best of circumstances, which these clearly were not, fought back.

"Mind your own business. I'll be the judge!"

"That's you . . . judge *and* jury for all occasions!"

Before long they were in a heated battle in the middle of the parking lot. That's when my father's anger hit a boiling point, the signal for my mother to back off. She slammed into the passenger seat and sat there steaming. Caught in the middle of their craziness, I instinctively took my mother's side.

"Dad," I said, my exhaustion at an all-time high. "Mom is just looking out for me. I've been through a lot and . . ."

My father threw up his hands, mumbling, "Well, it's a damn shame when you can't do anything to suit the women in this family. Get in the car!" And with that he grabbed the keys from me and jumped behind the wheel.

Later that evening at dinner, my father, still agitated, opened the conversation with his "I told you so" tone and things escalated from there. Trying to avoid confrontation, I did everything I could to keep from getting drawn into his web. Who was I kidding? I was no match for my father on a good day, let alone in my present condition. Within minutes I was engaged in a heated argument about my move to LA, my marriage to Scott and everything else he thought was wrong with me.

With my mother moving her silent treatment to the couch and giving his rage free rein, my father took full advantage. He worked his tirade until he had convinced me I was the complete and utter failure he perceived me to be. After several minutes of his pummeling, I found my voice and began my counterattack. But as my anger increased, along with the pitch of my voice, the dull ache in my breast intensified. Soon, with the pain hitting a ten on the pain meter, exhaustion overtook me. With no reserves left, I caved and began apologizing for everything I'd ever done to displease him. Drained and beaten, I excused myself and went to bed. He had made his point. Countless things were wrong with me and nothing was going to change that—not even the possibility of my dying from cancer.

Tossing and turning in bed, my heart in a million pieces, I wondered how much further down I would have to go. I reflected on the message the voice had given me about love and forgiveness. It seemed an impossible dream. How could I ever forgive this man for the hurt he continued to inflict?

As my body shut down, I welcomed the fatigue, hoping that sleep would rescue me from the pain in my heart. But my mind wouldn't let me sleep. It reminded me in no uncertain terms that my father had a right to be angry with me. I did deserve his wrath–look at the mess I'd made of my life. My mind concluded that maybe the only way out was to die. That way everyone could get on with life and I could finally find some peace.

The next morning I awakened from a restless sleep to find Scott sleeping beside me. As I gazed at his face, love and appreciation filled my heart. He was working so hard to support my healing, not to mention the supreme effort to get along with my parents. I was grateful he hadn't witnessed the previous night's fiasco, as I was sure he and my father would have come to blows. I vowed not to tell him about the fight, hoping with all my heart that I would ultimately make peace with my father and they could become friends.

The next day brought a welcome change of pace when the lab called with good news. My biopsy was negative, meaning my lymph was clear. As I hung up the phone, a tremendous relief swept over me, certain now that chemotherapy wouldn't be necessary. A little later Dr. K called to congratulate me on my lab results and asked me to set up an appointment to discuss our next steps.

"Steps, what steps?" I blurted. "My biopsy was clear!"

"Yes," he said. "And while this is wonderful news, Brenda, I still need you to see an oncologist." He went on to explain, "There is a new drug on the market, Tamoxifen, available to breast patients and I'd like you to discuss this with an oncologist."

He said it would help control estrogen levels. It wasn't until sometime later that I learned high levels of estrogen can be a major factor in the cause of breast cancer. As I listened to him drone on, my initial excitement turned to anxiety. When I realized he was not going to take no for an answer I agreed, on one condition.

"The appointment will have to wait until my parents leave. The stress of their visit along with the thought of talking to an oncologist . . . I just can't . . . "

"Say no more, Brenda. Let me put the nurse on and she can make an appointment for after their departure. Hang on."

Having decided not to mention this piece of information to my parents, they were excited to hear the all-clear. When Scott got up I told him in private the good and bad of what Dr. K had said. Feeling the same conflict of happiness and disappointment, we decided to count our blessings and celebrate the good news. Scott called in sick and the four of us spent a wonderful day together. Scott had the magical talent of always bringing a smile to my face and helping me forget my problems.

By the time my parents said their good-byes, I was more than ready for them to be gone. All week there had been a war going on inside me. Part of me wanted to patch things up with my father and share with both of them the truth about my current condition, while another part of me wanted to punish my father by keeping the details of my post-surgery follow-up hidden. By the end of the week the vindicator in me won and I sent them on their way without resolving my issues with Dad or telling them the truth about my recovery process. I somehow thought withholding from them would settle the score. Little did I know that I, not them, would be the one suffering from the pain of my guilt.

After they left I took a walk hoping to clear my head. Making my way up the street to a path I had walked many times, a strange sense began to overtake me. I was overcome with a throbbing pain on top of my head, then a flash of light, followed by the voice I'd been hearing for some time. It said if I were willing to let go of my need to be right, things with my father would change. But first a catch—I would have to forgive my father and myself if I wanted this to work.

Simultaneously, a powerful sensation was coursing through my body, bringing with it information about my needing to speak my truth. It said, "You must stand by your truth without feeling the need to defend yourself. What happened between your father and you is there to teach you to take a stand. To put an end to your need to be his victim so you may grow in love and forgiveness."

As this stream of consciousness flooded my mind and body, it was becoming clear to me that if I were willing to open my heart and release my negative judgments of my father, I could release his hold on me. And in the end, my health would greatly improve. Moments later, I found myself sitting on the ground wondering what had happened.

When I was able to get up and walk, I made my way home. But I was not the same woman who had gone for a walk to clear her head. Something profound had taken place. I was starting to grasp that the difficult situations in my life were opportunities to grow and change. I was being offered the opportunity to see things from a completely different perspective.

That evening as I wrote in my journal, there was no question something intense had happened that involved a simple piece of wisdom. A wisdom that gave new meaning to everything that had occurred in my life. And this voice? Deep in my soul I knew this divine presence was in fact Spirit calling me forth to shift my consciousness.

I was beginning to understand that my difficult circumstances were lessons in love. And I had a choice about how to respond to those lessons. I was also sensing that my thoughts, words, and deeds had an energetic effect on people. An effect that, like a boomerang, created energy that would come back to me in the form of good when I put out good and negativity when I put out negativity.

Over the next few days I read and reread what I had written in my journal. I recalled every detail of my epiphany while at the same time continuing to pray for the courage to follow these enlightened messages. I knew I had a long way to go before I would actually approach life from this enlightened place, before I would be able to open my heart to good.

Patterns run deep. It takes time, patience, and commitment to integrate a new way of thinking and being in our daily lives. Did I have what it would take to do this? I wasn't sure. But what I did know for sure was if I wanted to live a life of peace and good health, I was going to have to change. I was going to have to heal the negative patterns that were running my life because in my heart, I knew my time was running out.

10

Finding My Voice

After sitting in the oncologist's waiting room for half an hour, feeling I might pass out at any moment, I was finally ushered into his office. The room was dark and dingy, and though I'd caught a glimpse of a lovely grassy knoll right outside the window, the blinds were closed and a definite chill permeated the air. With the exception of some medical plaques there was no decoration on the walls. Even the black leather furniture reminded me of a funeral home. "God," I thought. "What have I gotten myself into?"

The longer I waited, the more my anxiety grew. Everything inside me screamed, *Get the hell out of here!* But before I could muster the courage to leave, Dr. C marched through the door thrusting his hand in my direction by way of introduction. He was a striking man with beautiful silver-white hair and an air of detachment. Once seated, he glanced at my paperwork and without looking at me began to talk about my case.

Addressing me by my married name he said, "Well Mrs. Warner, I read through your entire case history and after my conversation with Dr. K earlier today, it is our professional opinion that we start you on chemotherapy treatments on Monday. I suggest we do one session each week for six months starting with a light dosage, increasing the dose as your body adjusts. You pick the time. I'll have my nurse schedule it."

I was too stunned to speak. Somewhere between my conversation with Dr. K and this appointment, the two of them decided chemotherapy was what I needed. There wasn't even a mention of the drug

Tamoxifen. As far as they were concerned, this was a fait accompli. No alternative would be offered.

Struggling to quell the fear I felt might explode from my body, I held my tongue while he continued as if I weren't in the room. When he finally took a breath, I blurted out, "Wait! Don't I get a say in this? What about this new drug Dr. K told me about?"

Startled by my outburst he cut his monologue short and stared at me as if I were challenging every minute he had spent in medical school.

"Mrs. Warner," he patronized, "you must be sensible about this. You have a history of cancer. Your mother had uterine cancer and based on that and your own history, Dr. K and I determined it would be foolish of you not to move ahead with this treatment!"

"That may be," I said, trying to wrap my mind around what was happening, "but not without further thought and consideration about what I want."

As if I hadn't said a word he continued, "Nurse," he said into the phone, "please check the chemo schedule and work Mrs. Warner in ASAP."

I watched the scene unfold before me, dumbfounded at his deliberate dismissal of my concerns. I had heard stories from other cancer patients about this sort of behavior but couldn't imagine it was true. Now it was happening to me. I sat there enraged, unable to speak. Here I was again, his way or the highway. Would this forever be the pattern with the men in my life?

As he waited for his nurse to find some potential dates, he continued to shuffle through my paperwork. I sat in silence feeling I must be in a movie, someone else's movie.

Finally, my fight or flight kicked in. I jumped to my feet and headed for the door. My only thought, *There is no way I am going to listen to someone who is so completely out of touch with humanity.* I was a living, breathing human with a working brain. There was no way I was going to let this doctor intimidate me into doing something as serious as chemotherapy without further research and consideration.

Walking out the door I heard the theme music to *Rocky* in my head. Yes! I had just won my first bout! But my feeling of triumph was short-lived. Outside in the corridor, I connected the dots between this doctor and my father—controlling, dismissive and used to getting his way. Anger overtook me as I flashed back to one of my earlier insights. If I wanted to heal my body I had to heal the negative patterns that caused me to live in conflict and resistance. I had to forgive myself. I had to become the change I was seeking. A jumble of feelings engulfed me with guilt leading the pack. How could I have treated this doctor like that?

About to swallow my pride and return to offer an apology, the voice spoke, "Brenda, you must forgive yourself for your outburst and release your guilt. You need time to integrate these new ideas into your life."

She reminded me that until I could do that, my apology would be shallow. As I contemplated this, I became aware of the wisdom being communicated. Saying you're sorry doesn't mean much unless you are truly sorry. Releasing guilt is a process of forgiving the self, which calls for compassion and an open heart. I had a lot of work to do if I wanted to live this and not simply talk about it.

What I didn't fully understand was that life affords us lessons on a regular basis. Those lessons aren't meant to punish or diminish us but rather to show us where we are wounded and out of balance. With these lessons comes the opportunity to open our hearts, forgive ourselves and others, release what no longer supports our highest good, and heal patterns that keep us in a negative state. Only then can we move forward in a healthy, positive way.

The Universe in its loving perfection sends us what we need when we need it. When I was able to release my judgment about this doctor acting like an ass and fully grasp the lessons being offered, things began to make sense. He was not some enemy to be feared or scorned but rather a teacher on a long list of teachers I would encounter throughout my healing journey.

Digesting this information, it dawned on me that every person crossing my path was there to teach me something about myself, showing up at just the right moment to help unleash those lessons hiding deep in my subconscious. In other words, there are no accidents. Every person and experience was there for my good. My job was to see the truth, to stop blaming the outside world for my problems. If I could do this, if I could live this truth, I knew it would be a factor in regaining my health.

So, what was the lesson Dr. C was there to teach? It was no secret I had a lot of work to do around forgiveness. But as I considered this, my mind jumped in and hijacked my inner knowing. Maybe I should have listened to the oncologist's advice. Maybe I should begin chemo-therapy. In the space of a few minutes, the peace I was feeling had turned into fear and anxiety. Dr. K had told me what a skilled oncolo-gist Dr. C was. What was I doing? In a flash I was back to doubting myself, pushing aside the voice that had so consistently urged me to trust my inner knowing and once again giving in to the fear coursing through me.

By the time I reached home I was a mess, pleading with God to give me a sign, anything to let me know I'd done the right thing, refusing chemotherapy. Nothing came. Too distraught and exhausted to think about it anymore, I did what I always did. I said a million prayers and went to bed hoping that sleep would rescue me from my fear and self-doubt.

Waking a few hours later I remembered a dream. I was sitting in a cave across from a woman dressed in white. She was one of the most beautiful beings I had ever seen. She exuded love and light. As I sat basking in her beauty and warmth, she leaned forward and whispered something in my ear. In the moment I couldn't take in what she said. Later that evening, entering the details of the dream in my journal, her words came rushing back. And with her words came another surge of fear. Fear because I was being asked to trust myself. "It is time," I was told. "Time to stop doubting the knowing voice inside you."

The next day I called Dr. K to explain what had happened. "I was so uncomfortable. It just didn't feel right to me and I felt like I didn't have all the information I needed and I'm sorry but . . ."

"No Brenda, I'm sorry."

What? He was apologizing to me?

"Dr. C called me as soon as you left his office and explained you were resistant to our recommendations."

"I just felt I hadn't gotten all the information and . . ."

"No need to explain. I should have thought it through a bit more. I don't think Dr. C is the right choice of oncologist for you. Would you forgive me and agree to see another doctor?"

"No, no, no, no, no!" I screamed inside my head. "I don't want to see another doctor." That's not what came out of my mouth. "I guess I could," I mumbled.

"I have a much better choice for you," he explained. "Dr. R is very sensitive to his patients, always willing to hear their concerns. I realize that's something that is going to work much better for you."

"Really? And you didn't know this before you sent me to Dr. C?" That's what I should have said, but I didn't. I felt as if I were being tested. Was I considering seeing another doctor because I didn't want to disappoint Dr. K or was I going to stand my ground, politely refusing him? Ultimately, I was not strong enough to stand in my knowing. At the end of the conversation I acquiesced, agreeing to his request. He assured me I wouldn't be sorry. I was sorry already.

I felt angry with myself and guilty for being weak. I didn't know I was being given an opportunity to forgive myself. An opportunity to accept that I still had a long way to go before I could trust myself enough to speak my truth.

Since that time I've learned some things about higher knowledge. I've learned that when we say yes to its power, whatever stands in the way of our transformation will show up to be healed. In its divine wisdom, the Universe will provide plenty of opportunity to release our wounds so we may come alive to our authentic selves.

Two days later I found myself once again in a doctor's waiting room dreading my appointment. The only thing keeping me in my seat was my need to please Dr. K. It wouldn't be until later that I would look back and realize what a perfect demonstration this was of the power of my core beliefs. I was fully committed to the "please disease" and the role that fear played in making my decisions. It didn't matter that I knew better.

When Dr. R came in I was ready to steel myself to whatever he had to say. Thankfully there was a higher power at work that day. Dr. R turned out to be everything Dr. K said he was, sensitive to his patients and interested in their needs.

After formal introductions, he told me that having reviewed my records he was recommending that I *not* do chemotherapy.

"All things considered, I am convinced the drug Tamoxifen is a better choice for you."

What? What was he saying? Tamoxifen would be better? Honestly, all I heard was, "You don't need chemotherapy." That was enough for me. No further explanation necessary!

He went on to tell me how the Tamoxifen would be administered and how I would be monitored. He also said he would like to see me every three to six months depending on my progress.

"Your job," he said, "is to get plenty of rest and get on with your life."

I couldn't believe what I was hearing. This man, the head of oncology at one of the most prestigious hospitals in Los Angeles was telling me I didn't need chemotherapy. My intuitive voice had been validated. As the appointment wrapped up, I was bursting with joy. I couldn't wait to call Scott and tell him the good news.

He and I had been in agreement about chemotherapy treatments, convinced this protocol wasn't for me. At seventeen he had witnessed his father's rapid decline after chemotherapy and was sure the treatments had a lot to do with it. When I told him the good news he was thrilled that I wouldn't be risking that same fate.

Later that day, as I walked in the sun, I allowed myself to appreciate, for the first time in a very long time, how good it felt to be alive. I noticed the sky seemed bluer than usual, the sun brighter. "Finally," I thought. "Things are turning around."

That weekend Scott and I celebrated by going out. We called family and friends and told them the good news. They were happy but guarded as they felt I should reconsider chemotherapy just to be safe. But I was resolute. There was no way I was going to let their fear influence me. I had fought too hard for this higher ground and I was determined to stay there no matter what.

Dr. R set out my easy-to-follow routine. Every three weeks I would see Dr. K so he could examine my breast implant to ensure it was healing properly. Every three months I would go to Dr. R who would take my blood and chest X-rays to make sure the cancer wasn't showing up in my lungs. And once a year I was required to have a mammogram of my right breast. That was it.

With my confidence soaring, the weeks flew by. Before I knew it three months had passed. It was time for my first series of blood tests and X-rays, which confirmed I was making a solid recovery. Other than a few minor side effects from the Tamoxifen and some notable fatigue, Dr. K was pleased with my progress. He assured me that within a couple of months the side effects would pass.

While the following months were better than I expected, they weren't without their irritants. When I woke one day to my second yeast infection since starting the Tamoxifen, I called Dr. R to report it. He wasn't concerned since this was one of the many side effects of the medication. Even though I knew that, I was troubled that the medication didn't seem very effective and worried he was missing something. However, at my next check-up, my blood tests came back normal, so

Dr. K assured me there was no cause for alarm. But as this condition and the fatigue continued to plague me, I became haunted by the feeling there was something much deeper going on and I was the only one who knew it.

Having reached total frustration, I decided to try something. If the Tamoxifen was responsible for the infection and the fatigue, then it made sense to stop taking it until the infection passed. Knowing full well I would hear nothing but objections from Dr. R, I chose not to tell him.

Six months into my recovery I had my first chest X-ray and was given the all-clear. The infection had stopped but I was still battling fatigue so I decided to permanently discontinue taking the Tamoxifen. My hope was that over time my body would begin to regulate itself.

Nine months after surgery, I was starting to feel a bit better.

"I am pleased to hear that, Brenda," Dr. R beamed. "That is good news. The fatigue has lessened?"

"Actually, well, yes, it has."

"Is there something else?" he probed.

"I stopped taking the Tamoxifen."

"What?" he said cocking his head in disbelief.

"I stopped it." I said finding my voice. "It made me feel so bad all the time and it's hard to keep taking something you know is making you feel sick, so . . ."

"Brenda, that is unacceptable. This is not a game. These guidelines for your recovery are not optional. Do you want to recover?"

"Of course I want to . . ."

"Then you must follow the established procedure. This is not multiple choice. This is your life we're talking about."

"Right," I wanted to say. "*My* life, not yours, *mine*! *My* life, *my* choices."

But I didn't say that. I knew the only way to settle this was to let Dr. R think I would resume taking it. I didn't like lying to my doctor but I rationalized that being true to myself was more important than coming clean and having Dr. R at odds with me, so I shut my mouth and let him believe I was following protocol.

I also talked to him about my lack of sexual desire. He assured me that for some patients this is common after surgery. In time, he said, all of that would change. But for me, my inner voice was not satisfied and I left feeling he was missing something.

Scott and I had not discussed our lack of sexual intimacy and Dr. R suggested we do so. We had been so consumed with surviving this ordeal, both financially and emotionally, that my grief and our sex life had been pushed aside. After dinner that night, taking to heart what Dr. R suggested, I conquered my anxiety and opened the subject for discussion, hoping we would be able to have a meaningful dialogue.

"Scott," I started, "I just want to say I'm sorry I haven't felt much like being intimate. There have been so many distractions and I don't feel . . ."

"Don't worry about it, Brenda," Scott said, cutting me off. "I understand the problem. Really. It's not a big thing."

With that the conversation ended, leaving me with a sinking feeling he was keeping something from me. In recent weeks he had begun to pull away. He wasn't as affectionate as he had always been and we were no longer talking about our lives and what we wanted to accomplish.

When we were first together, we spent hours talking about our future and the dreams we wanted to fulfill. Now when I broached the subject, Scott would either guide the conversation in some other direction or act as though it wasn't important. Not really wanting to recognize the truth, that I was feeling this chasm between us, I went along.

This was one of my life patterns. When something unpleasant was staring me in the face, denial became my way of not exploring what needed to be explored. Fear drove every decision to deny and ignore the obvious. Fear's powerful force can keep us from moving forward, from facing that which begs our attention. When we choose to deny and ignore "what is," we live in resistance to what life is trying to teach us. Granted, facing our fears and having difficult conversations is not easy, but not doing so can lead to dire consequences, including health issues. I was the poster child for that!

The following months proved to be very difficult as Scott and I continued to grow apart, spending less and less time together. Powerless to do anything about our marriage, I became obsessed with my physical condition. With every ache and pain I feared the cancer was returning. I kept quiet hoping my silence would keep my worst nightmares at bay. I didn't realize this only exacerbated the already volatile terrain that had become my life. With my marriage on the rocks and cancer my reality, I found myself waiting. Waiting for the other shoe to drop. Waiting for the next crisis. Not a good place to be, as I was about to find out.

11

Premonitions

As the one-year anniversary of my surgery came and went, my condition remained much the same. In spite of doctor reports that maintained I was doing fine, nagging feelings that something wasn't right continued to vex me. The erosion of my energy, the awkwardness of living in this new body, and nightmares about losing my other breast persisted.

And while I was finally allowing myself to grieve the loss of my breast, I missed feeling feminine. I had always had a slender, toned body and was proud of the fact that I could eat anything and not put on weight. I also loved my breasts. Body image was a large part of my identity and that identity was being threatened.

For an actress there is tremendous pressure to look good. Now, adding to my lifelong battle with insecurity, I had the added anxiety of being disfigured. I was painfully aware that nothing was going to change that. Not even the implant surgery I'd had to rebuild what was lost could convince me I was okay. Outwardly I appeared normal but I was always uncomfortable with my many scars and a breast without an areola or nipple. To try and correct that would mean more surgery. Sooner or later I would have to accept I would never be physically "normal" again.

Navigating through the grief, anger, shame, and guilt when experiencing loss is extremely difficult. It doesn't matter if it's a body part, a loved one, or a job. Loss is loss. But through this process I learned when we deny our feelings, the results can be even more devastating.

Emotions, be they negative or positive, are meant to flow. Prolonged blocking of this flow weakens the body and taxes the immune system. Free-flowing energy is required for our bodies to stay healthy and vital.

But I was still entrenched in a medical model that treats symptoms, not the whole person. Nevertheless, on a subtle level things were happening. Messages were being imparted and received. At some point I knew my feelings would have to be dealt with even though I wasn't sure how I would go about it.

In addition to dealing with my illness every day, my heart ached. Scott was everything to me and I could no longer hide from the fact that we were rapidly growing apart. I had believed our relationship could weather anything. But who could have predicted what had become of our lives? As much as I tried to rationalize what was happening in our marriage, I couldn't escape the pain I felt. And though we never discussed it, I couldn't help but think Scott felt it too.

It wasn't surprising our relationship was low on the priority list. We were distracted, me with my illness, Scott with making money so we could survive. And truth be told, my distraction was not only about my illness but at times an even greater concern about how my body looked. I wasn't proud of my obsession with such a shallow concern and was aware it probably wasn't healthy but I couldn't help myself. Focusing on one part of the self, whether it's our bodies, our relationships, or our careers creates imbalance. Left unattended, that singular focus can create an unrealistic identity attachment.

It is an insidious process that supports the idea of separation between our inner and outer worlds and can spread . . . like a cancer. It shuts down our inner voice, separating us from our ability to tune into our intuition for guidance. Without intuitive guidance to instruct us, we lose the ability to make productive decisions or see solutions to our problems.

November arrived and with it came the loss of light that made me feel even more depressed. I also knew it was time to schedule a mammogram on my right breast. The inevitable phone call from Dr. R's office came. After scheduling my appointment, my mind started to spin a story about what I thought was happening. Soon desperation set in, followed by a full-blown panic attack. Looking for a way to escape my anxiety, I thought about calling Scott, but realized if I called him in my present condition I might freak him out, pushing him further away.

So, in a moment of lapsed sanity I picked up the phone and dialed my mother.

From the start, our conversation was rocky. I urged her past the small talk and shared with her how I was feeling about my upcoming mammogram. As soon as the words were out of my mouth, silence descended and I could feel her fear. For a moment we lingered in the quiet until I realized there was no way she was going to be able to offer the support I needed. This realization triggered my old pattern and I immediately went into caretaker mode making sure she was okay, disregarding my own needs.

Anger flared in me at her inability to respond the way I needed her to. I realized as long as I felt the need to rescue and support her, without asking that my needs be met, they never would be. With this thought, my anger dissipated and was replaced by sadness. I had been programmed to take care of everyone but me. And now, when I needed the love and support of my mom more than ever, it wasn't there and I didn't have a clue how to ask for it without feeling guilty.

I suddenly felt more alone than ever. Once again life was having its way with me, and no one, other than Scott, gave a damn. Not even my brothers whom I had only heard from once since my ordeal began. I shouldn't have been surprised. This was my family dynamic, and now, because I didn't know how to take care of myself, I was feeling the sting of the distance between us more than ever.

With my panic building, I had to do something to get away from the noise in my head. I decided to drive to Beverly Hills and go window-shopping. It was a destination I had purposely avoided since strolling those avenues only reminded me how poor we were. Acquiring the kind of wealth it would take to shop in the expensive stores that lined those streets was probably never going to happen. Out of sight, out of mind had been my protective stance. But that day I made an exception. For some reason it felt important to surround myself with beautiful things, to let the sights and sounds of shoppers on Rodeo Drive carry me to an alternate reality where I could indulge in my shopping fantasy.

Two days later I was standing in front of a mammogram machine that would expose if my breast tissue was healthy. As the nurse prepared me, I let my thoughts stray to how lucky I was to live in LA; how lucky to spend an afternoon window-shopping in Beverly Hills, filling my mind with anything to keep from thinking about what lay ahead.

Later as I was dressing, the nurse popped her head in and asked that I wait while the doctor reviewed my pictures. Alarm bells went off in my head and I began to pace back and forth, sure whatever was going on wasn't good.

After several torturous minutes, the nurse returned. "Mrs. Warner? The radiologist is ready for you."

I entered the room to find him, brows furrowed, standing in front of my pictures. "Mrs. Warner, I'm seeing an abnormality here on the lower part of your breast," he said pointing at the image. "It concerns me."

On high alert, all my senses engaged, my heart began to slow from its frantic pace. "Oh," I said, relief flooding through me, "that. That's nothing. Fifteen years ago a benign lump was removed so there's some scar tissue there. I forgot to mention it to the nurse."

"The scar isn't what I'm referring to. Look. See there?" he said zeroing in on the area in question. "There are three tiny specks below the dark mass that is your scar. They're calcium deposits."

Calcium deposits, I thought. *Well, that's nothing. Women get calcium deposits in their breasts all the time. Why is he being so reactionary?*

Continuing as if he'd heard my thoughts, "It isn't unusual for calcium deposits to show up in breast tissue but because of your history and because those deposits can sometimes be malignant, I'm very concerned about this presentation."

My body went cold while my face felt as if it were on fire. This can't be happening.

"I've already notified Dr. R's office and your pictures will arrive there later today. Don't worry. If he suspects a problem, you'll hear from him."

Don't worry? Did he just say, don't worry? With that he sent me on my way as if our business transaction was complete and all was in order.

Driving home my mind was going full force. Had my intuition been right? Was I going to lose my other breast? There would undoubtedly be another biopsy along with the possibility of another bout of cancer. My mind, like a broken tape recorder, was stuck in one place, accompanied by images of me even more disfigured. Thoughts of death and how this latest finding would once again impact my relationship with Scott took over.

During my first surgical procedure I had requested Dr. K biopsy my right breast just to be safe. He declined, saying nothing had appeared on my mammogram to warrant it. Nevertheless, I was concerned so I urged him to please run the test. But he was steadfast in his position and no biopsy was performed. Now, one year later facing the possibility of losing my other breast, I was mad as hell no one had listened to me.

By the time I reached my front door the phone was ringing. It was Dr. R.

"Brenda, I've just been reviewing your X-rays and I feel it's imperative we schedule a biopsy as soon as possible. I'm sorry to have to put you through this again but we really need to be on top of this."

Really, Dr. R? Really? That's pretty much how I felt when I asked you to biopsy it a year ago! Of course I didn't say that. I waited on the line while he transferred me to the nurse to schedule my biopsy . . . a year too late.

Getting off the phone, my mind was exploding as negative thoughts consumed me. My body began to expand and contract as if possessed by some alien life form. With each breath a sharp pain in my heart reverberated until I slumped to the floor, sobbing. After a couple of minutes the pain in my heart stopped but the pain in my soul remained. I was scared. I was alone. I was probably sick again. *Please,* I thought. *That's enough!*

When you're faced with life-threatening illness, nothing makes sense. Besides being terrified I was consumed with guilt and shame. I felt like a burden to Scott and a disappointment to my parents. I was also resentful—I resented my mother for being emotionally unavailable, my father for being so controlling and cruel, my brothers for their selfishness. And I was beginning to resent my doctors for not listening to me. Lastly, I resented God for deserting me. How could He allow the cancer to ravage my body like this? How could He take away my reproductive organs and now possibly both my breasts? And worst of all, why would He bring me this wonderful man I loved with all my heart only to lose him in this mess that had become my life?

Yet to discover that negative, unprocessed emotions are poisonous to the body, I dedicated myself to the way I was feeling. From my perspective, life had dealt me a bad hand. There was nothing I could do but hold accountable those responsible for my predicament.

"Why, God, are you punishing me and not them?" I screamed. When nothing came, I screamed louder. Finally, I heard a faint response say something about how God doesn't punish anyone—we do that to ourselves.

"Wait a minute," I retorted. "That's ridiculous!" Even though a tiny part of me thought this was probably true, at that moment it was more important to be right than to be enlightened. Someone must be blamed for my predicament. It certainly wasn't under my control.

I didn't know I had the choice to either take responsibility for my actions or be a victim. It never occurred to me I had been a *victim-volunteer* all my life. I wasn't aware I had given my power away to others, opening the door for people in my life to convince me I was someone other than who I really was. I found an odd comfort in my resentment of them for treating me with such disrespect, not realizing that all along I had been the one teaching them how to treat me.

We aren't born victims but we do have the choice to create situations that allow us to experience being a victim. And when we do, we simultaneously create the opportunity to evolve into more conscious beings as a result of what we learn from those victim experiences. We can believe we are victims, forfeiting our power to change our circumstances or we can use the lessons inherent in our victim mentality to advance our awareness. I had a ways to go before this awareness would integrate fully into my life, before I would be able to heal my anger and resentment, before I could forgive myself or others I believed responsible for my predicament.

Lying on the floor sobbing, I had an epiphany. This voice telling me things I wasn't ready to accept was kind, nurturing, and wise. Unlike the voice I had listened to as a child that was critical, dogmatic, unreasonable and made me feel bad about myself. As I contemplated this, I began to think maybe the voice from my childhood might be partially responsible for why I was sick. I realized that when I listened to it, negative feelings and thoughts took over making me feel less than, valueless and miserable. Surrendering to my altered state I heard, "Are you ready to release the negativity that has dominated your life?" "Yes!" I responded automatically without even thinking. "But how?"

As I waited for the answer, I was jolted back into the room by the ringing phone. It was Scott telling me he had the strangest feeling he should call. Chills ran up my spine as my entire being filled with love for him. Maybe some unknowable force was at work here. My fear of pushing him away kept me from reaching out and now here he was reaching out to me.

When I finished telling him what had happened he said, "I knew something wasn't right. I've been preparing myself all day for bad news." He paused. My heart skipped a beat. He took a deep breath and in that voice he used when he loved me the most, he said, "Brenda, whatever it is, whatever we have to face, we'll face it. We've done it before. We can do it again."

Over and over I would be reminded how talking things out, expressing what I was feeling never failed to make me feel better. And knowing I had Scott's support was always powerful medicine. I knew what I had to do next.

I got my mom on the phone and told her what had happened. When we were done, she insisted I tell Dad myself. "It's the least you can do for him," she said. My entire body went rigid. The least? *Well*, I thought. *Best not go there!*

"Brenda." The all too familiar tone that made me feel five again. "Dad."

He didn't take the news well and though he tried in his own way to be supportive, I could hear the underlying, "I told you so!" that permeated so many of our conversations. But instead of getting defensive, I thanked him for his concern. I thanked him, realizing that getting angry with him wasn't going to change my reality or make me feel better. After hanging up, having responded from a place of gratitude instead of blame, I noticed I felt lighter. Could there be some truth to what this voice was telling me?

As the day of my biopsy approached I was more and more on edge, finding it harder to stay positive and practice what I was learning. The night before my procedure, I dreamed I was sitting at the kitchen table where I had grown up, drawing pictures on a sheet of paper, when suddenly the lady in white appeared again. This time she spoke, asking me to write down what she was about to share and remember it always. Then she disappeared. When I glanced down at the paper, instead of the pictures I had been drawing, I saw words:

Each experience reveals your purpose.

Later that morning when Scott walked in the door, he looked at me curiously and said, "What is going on with you? Something's happened."

When I finished telling him about the dream, he responded, "I don't know what that all means, exactly, but I have always felt something beyond the cancer has been trying to get your attention."

Vibrating with what he said, I didn't trust myself to respond. I felt as if I were bridging two worlds: the world I had known where fear and insecurity were my constant companions and this new world that beckoned to me with love and support.

Before crawling into bed he reminded me, "It's time to stop doubting yourself. Start trusting what's coming through." And as he drifted off to sleep he said, "In time everything will make sense."

Taking his words to heart I realized how many times I had sabotaged myself. How many times I had discounted the messages coming through, allowing myself to slip into fear and negativity. Maybe it was time to surrender to this guidance, to trust. Maybe the cancer was trying to awaken me to some part of myself I didn't know. Maybe it was there to help me find a purpose beyond my illness. For now, all I could do was wait.

Part Three

Holding the High Ground

12

The Face of Betrayal

Arriving at the hospital, Scott and I entered the all too familiar scene: mountains of paperwork to fill out and the endless wait for Dr. K. When he finally appeared we were armed and ready. We had questions and we wanted answers.

The main question was what he thought of my mammogram. Much to our surprise, he told us he was fairly optimistic. From what he could tell, the white specks appeared to be calcium deposits and nothing more. He answered our questions and explained the biopsy procedure assuring me it would be an easy process, not more than a couple hours. Being a veteran of several surgeries and one other biopsy, I had my doubts about how easy the procedure was going to be. I insisted he tell us exactly what he was going to do.

"I'll use the mammogram as a guide to locate the calcium deposits and insert a hollow needle into your breast. Then I'll push a plastic line filled with dark-colored dye through the center of the needle so I can mark the infected area. This will make it possible for me to see where to cut into the tissue. I'll remove the needle but leave the plastic line so I can see where to do the extraction without doing excess damage to the surrounding area. We'll do all this with a local, only using an anesthetic during the actual cutting."

Listening to his explanation, I was reminded that doctors and patients have entirely different perspectives of what constitutes an easy procedure!

Once Scott and I were alone in the room, he became very quiet. Glancing over at the love of my life, it hit me—this past year had really taken a toll on him. He had aged ten years and though he never let on, I knew he was fighting his own internal battles. I felt closer to him than I had in a long time but still wondered if we would ever be able to address all the pain and financial distress this disease had brought into our lives. Would it be possible for us to restore our marriage?

Cancer can exhaust a family. It can create havoc financially, emotionally, spiritually, and as in my case, sexually. Although there was the possibility my body would eventually heal, I didn't know if it was possible to heal from the debris the cancer would leave in its wake.

Both lost in our own thoughts, I didn't notice the nurse's presence until she was wheeling me out of the room. I glanced over at Scott and saw him wink at me with his endearing "don't worry, everything will turn out fine" look, but in my heart of hearts, I knew things were anything but fine. How were we going to pay for this procedure? And what in God's name would we do if Dr. K found cancer again?

I had been given the choice of being awake with a local anesthetic or being knocked out. Wanting to hear what was being said once Dr. K reached the calcium deposits, I opted to remain awake. Cutting into my breast tissue he said it looked healthy. I was incredibly relieved but knew the official biopsy results would be the final word. Nevertheless, based on his observation I felt hopeful. The procedure complete, I went back to my room to wait for the results.

Forty-five minutes later, Dr. K walked through the door interrupting a great conversation Scott and I were having about our future. For the first time in a long time we felt hopeful. I would get my acting career off the ground. Maybe Scott and I could even work together. We were finally on the road to fulfilling the reasons we had moved to LA.

As we turned to see Dr. K enter the room, our excitement turned to dread. One look at his face told us everything we needed to know.

He took my hand as he explained. "Brenda, Scott," he said, making eye contact with each of us, "the lab found malignant cells in your tissue. I'm afraid there's going to be further surgery required."

He took a deep breath as if bracing himself for something more. I knew what it would be before it came out of his mouth.

"Brenda, I'm so sorry. We aren't going to be able to save your . . ."

"I know," I interrupted, not trusting myself to hear him say the words.

So, there it was—the reason I had felt so exhausted for the past year. My body wasn't recovering. It had been fighting cancer all along. I felt as if I would explode.

Betrayal, anger, grief poured out of me as I shouted, "What about all the blood tests? What about all that talk about how nicely I was recovering? With all the tests you did, why didn't you know?"

Fighting back his own tears, Dr. K offered us a few minutes alone before any further talk about scheduling another surgery. Once he was out of the room, Scott pulled me into his arms. We held on for dear life, knowing the road ahead was anything but certain.

There are no words to fully describe my feelings that day. In a matter of minutes I went from happy and hopeful to helpless and powerless. Holding each other, letting the tears flow, something we hadn't done together in a very long time, my heart ached for Scott. Here we were a year later right back where we started. But this time with a high probability that my situation was even more serious than before. When Dr. K returned, we were in no condition to make any decisions about anything. We agreed on a surgery date and left it at that. Any other details would have to be worked out once we could think again.

By the time we arrived home my grief had spun me into a state of devastation. I went into the bathroom and locked the door. I was desperate to escape the pain I was feeling, desperate to find a way to quell my fear. But it wasn't until I stopped resisting that I was able to take a breath, allowing a sliver of truth to hit me.

In that moment, my dream and the words I had written came rushing back. *Remember to look for the meaning behind this.* What meaning? No, I was in too much pain, too much conflict to look for the meaning. The more I thought about this, the more agitated I became. Didn't God understand my life was falling apart? That the last thing I wanted to do was search for meaning? Didn't He know it was going to be hard enough to face the fact I had cancer again, much less find some obscure mystical meaning in all of this? Obviously He did not!

The days that followed were torture. I vacillated between anger and desperation. My soul felt dead. My inner voice was silent. My heart hurt and nothing Scott said or did could help me as I continued to withdraw into self-pity. My mind urged me to pull myself together. *Be strong,* was its mantra. *No matter what,* my mind kept repeating, *get through this with strength and dignity.*

Back on my pre-surgery schedule, there were a number of necessary tests including a bone scan and chest X-ray. But before having those done, I made an appointment to see my oncologist. I wanted to find out why he hadn't been aware I still had cancer.

Arriving at his office I was ready to let him have it. But he was in his own preemptive mood.

"Brenda," he explained, "with many cancers, the disease often has to reach advanced stages before a tumor is apparent. In other words, by the time cancer is discovered, it can be too late to do anything about it."

This seemed impossible to me.

"With the billions of dollars spent on cancer research every year," I demanded, "how can there not be a more efficient way of tracking this disease?"

"Unfortunately, better ways of early detection have simply not been developed yet."

As our conversation wound down, he apologized for not realizing the severity of my condition sooner. He assured me he had done his best to track my illness but our conversation did little to quell my anger or put to rest all my questions. I was disgusted with conventional medicine for not having the answers and as much as I respected Dr. K, I was disgusted with him too.

And so it was with this frustration raging through me that I made my next stop, the hospital. I was armed and dangerous, intent on making my doctors realize their medicine was falling short and somebody needed to take responsibility.

Upon completing my chest X-rays, I was instructed to wait in the dressing room for the results before reporting for my bone scan. It was an all too familiar scene that did nothing to ease my already foul mood. Thirty minutes passed and I was still waiting.

"Excuse me," I called to a nurse passing by. "Do you know what is going on?"

"I'll see what I can find out," she said, barely slowing her pace.

Ten minutes later she returned. "Your X-rays have been given to the radiologist for review. As soon as he's had a chance to go over them, I'll come get you."

God please, I thought, *this can't be happening again!* Another twenty minutes went by.

Poking her head in my room, the nurse called to me. "The radiologist is ready to see you."

I walked into yet another sterile hospital room where I was met with yet another emotionally disconnected doctor who explained that the picture of my left lung revealed a shadow.

"This could indicate trouble." He droned on, "Shadows on an X-ray usually indicate cancer on the lung. Based on what I'm seeing, I'm going to send your pictures to your surgeon and oncologist for their opinion. In the meantime," he instructed, "remain calm."

He did not just say that to me. My head was spinning. He instructed his nurse to do another set of X-rays on my left lung and then prepare me for a cat scan so he could get a better look. With that he dismissed me.

I followed the nurse to the X-ray lab. When my X-rays were completed, I was taken to another section of the building where I was left in a cold, dark room to wait for my cat scan.

"The doctor will be with you shortly," the nurse assured me.

But shortly in hospital talk is a relative term. Another thirty minutes went by before the radiologist made his entrance. Another thirty minutes to spin the tale of not only breast cancer ravaging my body, but now, lung cancer as well.

The radiologist, true to his earlier lack of compassion, didn't apologize for keeping me waiting, nor did he take a moment to assuage my fears. Instead, in his most professionally detached tone he told me what was going to happen. I was trembling as the steel machine hovered over me like an alien probe, scanning my body for signs of impending death. I anxiously awaited some discourse from him telling me what he was seeing, but he was silent. After several torturous minutes, he spoke.

"Well, Mrs. Warner, this is very interesting. I don't see a thing." He then excused himself and walked out the door.

Before I could respond, before I could ask one question, he walked out the door, leaving me propped up on the table like a piece of meat. A few minutes later he returned.

"It appears the technician made a mistake while taking the first set of X-rays. From what I can determine there is no shadow, no cancer."

With that, he instructed his nurse to take me down the hall for my bone scan and made his exit. I was too stunned to speak. But as things began to sink in, I became enraged! My mind went on a tirade!

How dare he put me through hell for over two hours and then act as if having metastasized breast cancer was no big deal? I could not comprehend his behavior. He had simply sent me on my way as if nothing had happened. My mind was a jumble of questions.

What had become of bedside manner? Was it merely a quaint concept of old? How do people get to the point of not caring? How could you stray so far from your heart that you no longer allow yourself to care about others? Is this the new modern medicine? And if so, how can healing occur in this environment? People are not statistics! People are human beings and deserve to be treated with respect, honor and compassion.

I climbed off the machine and dressed as fast as I could. "I need to get this bone scan done now, immediately," I stated in no uncertain terms.

"I'm sorry, Mrs. Warner, but we're not ready for you quite yet," the nurse said, hedging the situation.

"Then I'm leaving," I said as I made my way to the door. "I've waited long enough."

With that, she guided me down the hall. I burst through the doors into the lab, startling the technician, and hopped on the table.

"I need to have this test done and it needs to be done now."

"And you are?" asked the technician with one eyebrow raised.

"This is Mrs. Warner," my attending nurse replied as she scurried into the room behind me.

"Well, Mrs. Warner," the technician began in her most patient and condescending voice, "that's not how we do things around . . ."

She was interrupted by the nurse whispering in her ear. I don't know what she said but I had a pretty good idea based on the fact that twenty minutes later, the test completed, I walked out the door.

Fleeing the hospital, I swore I would never go through that again. What was the world coming to? My life was falling apart and no one seemed to notice or care! And though I failed to see that what I was experiencing held yet another opportunity for me to take the high road, I had at least honored my feelings, expressing my anger and not kowtowing to the doctors and medical attendants as I had before. It may not have been the most constructive road but in my own way

I had taken charge of the situation. I didn't sit by pretending to be okay with what was happening and for that bit of self-expression, I felt good.

Throughout my healing process, I learned the hard way that taking charge of my life was a very important step in dealing with my cancer. From an emotional standpoint, a big part of the root cause of this disease stems from swallowing your feelings, hiding your truth from yourself and others, giving your power away, trying to please others by seeking their acceptance and approval.

Lacking the confidence or awareness to take a stand on my own behalf, I had repeatedly been unable to stand up for my truth. I felt disempowered and vulnerable. It wasn't until later in my recovery that I came to understand this was the issue at the core of what angered me. It was my behavior that fostered resentful feelings in me, threatening to make my illness worse.

After sharing my experience with Scott, he suggested I call Dr. K and tell him what had happened. I chose not to because I felt like I was always complaining. Understanding my dilemma, Scott offered to make the call.

That afternoon I received a call from Dr. K, "I am so sorry, Brenda, that you had to go through that. I'm sure it was frustrating and difficult for you but we have a lot coming up. Let's try and let go of what happened today and focus your energy on the surgery. I promise you I will speak to the doctors and nurses involved and make sure this never happens again."

After our conversation, I felt somewhat vindicated. I promised I would do my best to get past my feelings and stick to what was important. Later, as I contemplated what had happened, I realized it is one thing to be conscious of your anger and express it, but something altogether different to let your anger consume you, becoming your entire focus.

The next morning Scott and I made the trek to the hospital. While I was still feeling overwhelmed from the events of the day before, I made up my mind that no matter what happened, no matter what the doctors found or recommended, there would be no more surgeries and no chemotherapy—even if it meant losing my life!

That afternoon, Dr. K surgically removed my right breast and extracted fifteen lymph nodes. As before, the nodes were sent to the lab for analysis and as before we would wait for the results. My stay at the hospital was uneventful and within two days I was back home awaiting my test results. In the meantime, Scott continued to work and I, completely exhausted from my ordeal, did nothing but sleep.

Four days later Dr. R called. "Brenda, your biopsy indicates there was cancer present in four of your nodes. I'm sorry to have to tell you this but please know how lucky you are the cancer was detected before it traveled through all of your nodes."

Lucky? Funny, I didn't feel lucky. Not only did I have cancer again but now the cancer had invaded my lymph, stealing not only my breast, but also my hope.

13

Honoring My Intuition

Two days after receiving my biopsy results, I went to see Dr. R. Scott and I were still convinced chemotherapy was not a viable choice for me. Most of our friends and family didn't agree. Determined to not let them sway me, I had to admit a small part of me was still a little uneasy with my decision. Even so, I felt it was time to trust my intuition. Convincing Dr. R of this would be another matter. Knowing it's time to go against the model is one thing, confronting an expert with your conviction when it's based on a *feeling* rather than facts is quite another. This was going to be a real test for me in honoring my truth.

Scott contacted Dr. Lewis, a chiropractor friend of his in Seattle who was part of a network of holistic doctors. Dr. Lewis referred us to Dr. Gonzalez, a New York MD of Immunology who also offered an alternative approach specializing in treating cancer, particularly breast cancer. In checking him out, we discovered he was in good standing with the American Medical Association and decided to forward my medical records to see if I was a good candidate for his program.

After speaking with his nurse, I noticed that for the first time in a long time I felt focused and peaceful—a feeling that told me I was on the right track. I was very impressed with the questions his nurse asked and even more impressed when she shared that she too had had breast cancer and been told she had three months to live, fifteen years earlier. She had been a patient of Dr. Gonzalez and after her recovery had gone to work for him. I was now sure we were on the right track.

The next day was my scheduled follow-up with Dr. R. Based on the information I'd gotten from Dr. Gonzalez's nurse, I was armed with a list of questions. But before I had a chance to get to them, Dr. R, well aware of my objections to chemotherapy, presented his prognosis.

"Brenda, I know we've had our differences about some of your treatment, but I would be remiss if I didn't give it to you straight." Hunkering down for the bottom line, he continued. "It is my best professional opinion that within one to three years, and let me stress that three years is stretching it, there is a very good probability your cancer will metastasize."

"What does that mean, exactly?" I asked, ready to refute his learned opinion.

"What it means, exactly, is that it will spread to your bones, brain, or lungs," he answered, boring into my eyes. "Please understand, this is not a big stretch. It is a very predictable prognosis for many women who have had breast cancer." He waited for me to say something but I was not prepared to go head to head with him. I sat silently, his invitation to continue.

"Let me add, Brenda," he warned, "if that happens, there is a very high probability that at that point, chemotherapy won't be much help. On the other hand, if you do chemotherapy right away, you will have a chance of living at least five years, maybe more."

This was my prize? *Maybe* five more years? Five more years of being sick? Five more years of feeling like hell? Five more years of waiting for the other shoe to drop? Was this the best I could hope for? The best modern medicine had to offer?

"Can you guarantee me at least five years if I do your protocol?" I asked, my certainty about not doing chemotherapy starting to wane.

"I'm afraid not, Brenda. No one can give you a guarantee," he said, trying to soften the blow. "And let me add this: if you refuse this treatment, the probability of your cancer metastasizing within a year is high. And if that happens, you probably won't make it."

As I listened to his words of doom, my worst fears came to the surface and once again, I began to question myself.

Recognizing this, he said, "Before you make any concrete decisions, talk it over with Scott. But," he cautioned, "I urge you to make your decision quickly. It is imperative that you begin treatment right away."

By the time I reached home, my desperation was once again in the driver's seat. My first instinct was to call a couple friends and seek their opinions. Once I had that information I would act on the majority vote, as if they somehow knew better than I. But this time something inside urged me to trust my original feelings.

All along, the guidance I had been receiving was to look within for answers. To make my own decisions, trusting that whatever decision I made, no matter how difficult it seemed, would be right for me. Discussing what I had learned that day with Scott, he was still in favor of my following my intuition, but he understood my dilemma and after hearing what Dr. R had said, agreed to support me no matter what I decided.

Prayer had become a big part of my life. I asked God to give me peace in my decision. I wanted to be able to move ahead without fear dictating my every move. Surrounding myself with a prayerful energy, I was feeling much more serene. That night, I slept better than I had in some time and in the morning awoke still at peace.

Later that day, when the information I requested from Dr. Gonzalez arrived, I dove into it with abandon. I was eager to read it before making my final decision, hungry to know all I could about this program. When I finished the material, one thing stood out. This program was designed to *assist the body in healing itself while focusing the patient's attention on wellness, not disease.* Here it was, in black and white, the answer to my prayers.

As a final confirmation, I needed to complete one last step to be absolutely sure of my decision. Taking several deep breaths, I centered myself. With gentle focus I was finally able to drop into a deep place within that I had never connected to before. Centered in that place, I asked if this program was what my body needed to heal. Within moments my body was flooded with a sense of loving warmth. After allowing myself to bask in this feeling for a while, I went on to ask if chemotherapy was what my body needed to heal. I immediately felt as though there was a clenched fist sitting in the middle of my stomach. That's when I knew for sure I had found my program.

This may sound simplistic, and in many ways it is simple, but not easy. The expanse from the brain to the heart, though short in distance, is one of the longest roads we travel on the way to trusting our own intuition.

It took a while to get up my nerve to call Dr. R and inform him of my decision. But once I had him on the phone, it turned out to be a much easier conversation than I had anticipated.

"I know it will not come as a surprise to you that I am not in favor of this decision but it is your decision," he offered.

"I know that," I said, relieved that after all we'd been through together, our last conversation would not be contentious.

He went on to inform me, "I will no longer be responsible for you as my patient."

"I understand completely. And I want to thank you for your help and support."

Putting the receiver down, I instantly felt relieved and confident of the direction I had chosen.

There hadn't been one time in my life I could remember feeling confident about my decisions. Fear had always stopped me. This time was different, not because I was fearless but rather because I had decided to push through my fear and honor my inner voice.

Scott was thrilled to hear the news and suggested it might be a good idea to talk with some of Dr. Gonzalez's patients. We called his office and asked for references. His nurse was happy to accommodate and gave us a list of past and current patients who had consented to speak with potential patients. That evening we called as many as we could. We were delighted to find that they were enthusiastic, upbeat and for the most part, doing very well.

The next order of business was to call family and friends to let them know my decision. Once again true to the established pattern, they were skeptical but also curious about my enthusiasm and certainty for Dr. Gonzalez's program when I knew so little about him and his work. For me, the answer was simple. I was finally following my intuition. I trusted that this program and Dr. Gonzalez had entered my life at the perfect moment. They claimed they understood, but Scott and I could feel their hesitancy through the phone lines.

Right before the Christmas holidays, I received a call from Dr. Gonzalez's nurse informing us that after reviewing my case, the doctor was sure his program could help me. They had scheduled us to begin right after the holidays. In light of what my oncologist had expressed to us about the urgency of treatment, this took us by surprise. But when I went to my heart, it felt right. So, we decided to relax over the holidays and do our best to put the events of the past year behind us.

When we told my parents there was no urgency for me to go to New York until after the holidays, they offered to fly us home for

Christmas. Our first inclination was to decline, but after giving it some thought, we felt it could be the perfect time to share this program with them and hopefully put them at ease with my decision.

During our visit the subject of intuition came up a few times. Everyone was curious about how I was able to make such an important decision using only my intuition. With this approach still fairly new to me, I found it somewhat difficult to explain that I used meditation, feelings, and a knowing that came through to guide me. I wanted to share about the "voice" I had been hearing, but quickly realized that might be a mistake. It would only make them think I was crazy.

Since my parents were Christians, they wanted to know where God fit into this. I did my best to explain that this was, in and of itself, the inner knowing I had spoken to them about before. And even as I tried to explain, I knew enough to know that unless they had already found this source within themselves, this spiritual concept would probably be impossible to grasp. I understood their cynicism. I knew how long I had struggled to find and trust my own inner voice.

We are raised in a society where we learn to trust in experts and things outside ourselves. I knew by many people's definition I would be considered crazy for going against expert advice. But my decision was not about being logical or going with the status quo. My decision was about seeking a higher guidance and honoring that guidance to the best of my ability.

I had hoped we could all come together in harmony but I was also fully aware that most of their speculation and doubt was never clearly voiced. No one was willing to say forthrightly what he really thought. But I knew instinctively that almost everyone believed I was committing suicide. And though this was disappointing, Scott and I completely understood and accepted they were incapable of fully embracing my choice.

I would learn later in my treatment with Dr. Gonzalez that one of the important aspects of his program is the need for the patient to have unconditional support from family and friends. If that is not in place, the patient is asked to eliminate those negative influences during the recovery process. That is not to say those relationships must be cut out forever but it is his belief that for the patient's wellbeing it is necessary to eliminate them during healing.

Though doing this felt a little threatening to me, the nurse explained that it was very important to begin letting go of "toxic relationships." She described those to mean "any relationships that were controlling, angry, guilt-ridden, hateful, manipulative, or negative for any reason." Dr. Gonzalez believed that a patient's recovery involves being in a safe, loving, supportive environment that is conducive to healing. Family, spouses, and friends can have a great influence on one's life, so if people are negative for any reason, they can have a detrimental effect on the patient. I knew exactly what he meant.

It was imperative that I rethink everything about my life. Looking at my relationships, it was easy for me to see that many of them had been emotionally and spiritually toxic. If I was going to commit myself to getting well, I had to be willing to commit to changing or eliminating the relationships that weren't serving me.

As our visit home came to an end, I realized I had made it through an entire week without arguing with my father. Scott and I assumed my mother must have cautioned him not to push his opinions on us during this vulnerable time and for once, he must have listened. It was truly wonderful being with him when we weren't at each other's throats.

The morning we left I said a prayer of thanks for being given this reprieve with my father. I knew the peace between us was not likely to last but nevertheless I left that day with gratitude in my heart and a sense that once again, my life was about to change in ways I couldn't imagine.

14

Ready or Not

I sometimes think it is a perverse law of nature that the Universe provides us with the lessons we need when *it* feels we are ready, whether we feel ready or not. I had come a long way but after initially returning home from my parents' refreshed and ready to take on what awaited in New York, my mind started its familiar dance. It conjured every negative, self-defeating story it could to erode my self-confidence and return me to a depressive state. It repeatedly informed me this program was never going to work for me and what's more, Dr. Gonzalez didn't feel I was a good candidate after all.

It was during this time I became acutely aware how hard it is to break old patterns. It occurred to me how valuable it would be if I could catch those negative reactions so ingrained in me before they threatened to wear a permanent groove in my psyche. Maybe even perform a preemptive strike on my knee-jerk responses and make a different choice. I knew this would be easier said than done. I also knew things had to change if I stood a chance of reclaiming my health. So, on the heels of this revelation I recommitted to meditation and prayer knowing these disciplines would help me stay centered and positive.

I also discovered a side benefit I hadn't anticipated. When I became cognizant of my responses and chose a more positive reaction, the Universe supported me in kind, sending messages of love and support. These messages came as reminders to be patient with myself, not to expect too much—a message my perfection-addicted consciousness surely needed. I was being shown that the more loving I was willing to be with myself, the more peace and wellbeing I would experience in my world.

I still had my ups and downs but when I consciously gave myself permission to experience my feelings, I found the emotions that in the past took over my life, subsided. I was in recovery from a set of self-imposed rules that, for years, had held me hostage to completely unrealistic standards. This process was not about being perfect or achieving a quick fix. This was about healing my life so I could heal my body.

On the day we were scheduled to leave for New York, my body once again demanded my attention. Because I had worked so hard to get back to the centered feeling my soul craved, I was surprised to wake with an upset stomach. Traveling was the last thing I wanted to do. Was I creating yet another roadblock? We knew we couldn't postpone this trip or my treatment any longer. I had to make the best of it.

After taking something for my stomach, we made our way to the airport and boarded the red-eye to New York. The flight wasn't full so I was able to get a seat in the back of the plane where I could lay down. But in spite of this prone position, my mind continued to rage, making sleep impossible. Once again, all the work I had done seemed to be slipping away. Had I made the right choice?

The following day, standing in front of Dr. Gonzalez's office door, I was immobilized. I had come all this way, I wanted to do this program but I couldn't move. As much as I had been looking forward to our meeting, I was finding it difficult to get past the negative scenario I had created in my imaginary conversation with the doctor.

Digging deep to find my courage and breathing into my fear, I opened the door and walked into the waiting room. My heart stopped. Sitting in front of me were five patients waiting to see Dr. Gonzalez. I was horrified at how pale, thin, and incredibly fragile they looked. I had never seen people who looked so close to death. The scene went right to the core of all my fears.

With my confidence on a rapid downhill slide, I again questioned my decision to come. I tried my best to stop staring at everyone but there was one woman whose aura haunted me. She appeared to be in her early forties, fairly tall from what I could tell, and probably weighed less than a hundred pounds. Her skin was gray, her eyes sunken deep into their sockets. Seeing this physical reality so close up reminded me how devastating cancer is to the human body and why some people choose to give up rather than carry on.

As I obsessed over her condition, I prayed this wasn't going to be my fate. I could feel Scott's uneasiness, but sensing I was scared enough for both of us, he reached for my hand, squeezing it to let me know we were in this together.

When the time came for us to meet Dr. Gonzalez, he came to the waiting room to greet us. I was taken aback at how young and handsome he was. Although he maintained an air of professionalism, there was a warmth about him that eased some of my doubt.

"Mrs. Warner? Mr. Warner? Welcome. Let's go in back and have a chat."

Once seated in his office, he began, directly and to the point.

"I have gone over your records extensively, Mrs. Warner. Having received your medical information as well as your mammograms and the results from the hair sample testing, I have been able to determine a myriad of things."

I became acutely aware I wasn't breathing. *Is there any air in this room?* I thought.

"Through your testing we've measured how much active cancer is in your body and what mineral deficiencies you have. I won't sugarcoat it—your cancer rate is quite high."

This "chat" was not helping my airflow. I became aware that Scott was also holding his breath. Was my worst-case scenario coming true? Was I not a candidate for this program? Time seemed to stand still until Dr. Gonzalez spoke again.

"But," he offered, "I do feel this program will be able to help you."

With the good news spoken, Scott and I both let out our collective breath and were able to focus more fully on what the doctor was saying.

"A large part of this program consists of cleansing routines to rid the body of toxins. There is also an extensive regimen of vitamins, minerals, enzymes, and organic raw foods. From your tests I've determined which diet would be best for you to correct your particular vitamin, enzyme, and mineral deficiencies."

I'd heard the term "organic raw foods" before but didn't really know what that meant. He explained it is food grown in soil that isn't chemically fertilized, sprayed with insecticides and/or defoliants, or otherwise treated with chemicals or radiation.

He went on to explain, "It is my belief that many cancers, particularly breast cancer, are caused by an overload of toxins in the body as a result of exposure and/or ingestion of chemicals and poisons."

As he continued through my medical history, he told us why he felt I was predisposed to cancer. Having grown up in Eastern Washington I had been exposed to radiation from the Hanford nuclear site. Between 1947 and 1951, radiation leaks were a daily occurrence. As a result, the air, water, and soil were polluted. Even though we lived many miles from the site, the radiation was carried downwind, blanketing several counties in that area.

Although Dr. Gonzalez couldn't prove his theory, he felt strongly this had something to do with my condition. The fatty tissue in breasts tend to store chemicals and toxins, making them susceptible to disease.

"But," he went on, "let me add, I absolutely believe a person's mental, emotional, and spiritual attitude have a great deal to do with the condition of their health."

I felt an odd relief to hear him say this, for as much as I originally didn't want to accept it, what he said confirmed what I had come to believe was true for me.

"And before I let you go, let me also emphasize the importance of you giving your body every opportunity to heal by resting and listening to its signals. I guarantee you will need every ounce of energy to create the optimum environment for your body to heal. With that in mind, you will not be exercising at all for the first three months. Eventually," he went on, "as you show positive results, we'll incorporate walking into your program."

We spent two hours with Dr. Gonzalez that day and while we were overwhelmed with the information, we were also impressed with his knowledge. No other doctor had mentioned any of the possible links he discussed with us as contributing factors to cancer. We left that afternoon with a different perception of what constitutes healing and what it means to be truly healthy. My confidence was flying high and I was excited about the direction my life was taking.

Scott, fascinated with the information Dr. Gonzalez had shared, asked if there was anything he could read about it. Dr. Gonzalez gave him a manuscript he had written based on the research of Dr. William Kelly, a colleague with whom he had studied for many years. Dr. Kelly's program targeted pancreatic cancer patients, showing remarkable success with this usually fatal disease.

Dr. Kelly was a dentist who based his work on what he termed *Metabolic Ecology*, the study of balancing the body through nutrition, vitamins, minerals, enzymes, detoxification, and rest. The program is designed to create an environment in which the *body can heal itself*. Scott stayed up all night reading and by morning was convinced we were on the right track.

The next day we returned for my physical check-up and a printout of the program Dr. Gonzalez had designed for me. Glancing through it, I realized life would never be the same. For one thing, my entire diet was about to shift dramatically. For at least the next year I would be eating a diet that consisted of raw organic fruits and vegetables, nuts, whole grains and organic raw calf's liver. The program also required that I drink a quart of organic carrot juice each day, along with a tablespoon of flaxseed oil. Things that were absolutely forbidden were dairy, meat, caffeine, sugar, soft drinks, processed or canned foods and deserts of any kind. Studying the diet I began to get a picture of my days filled with juicing, detoxifying, mega-doses of pills and boring food. Though it seemed a lofty assignment, I knew enough at this point to know I had two choices: change my lifestyle completely or risk becoming a statistic. I hadn't come this far for the latter choice. An increasingly clearer picture of the reality of my situation prepared me for what was sure to be a challenging ordeal.

Finished with my physical exam, Dr. Gonzalez asked if we had any questions. I started out by asking if I could cheat on the program and still get well. Dr. Gonzalez's eyes flashed as he leaned forward and said forcefully, "Brenda, you have a serious illness. I'm not going to tell you, you can't cheat. But if you are not 100 percent committed to getting well, you won't. So, make up your mind and tell me now."

With that he leaned back in his chair awaiting my response. I got it! Cancer is serious business. He expected his patients to honor the responsibility of regaining their health. Having been called out, I hesitated to ask my next question, but knew if I left his office without getting all the information I needed, I would be sorry.

So, I took a deep breath and asked him, "Do you feel your program will work for me?"

Smiling, he explained, "While you aren't as sick as some of my patients, your success depends a lot on your motivation." He went on, "Often the sicker the patient, the more motivated they are. Consequently the sicker patients sometimes do better than some of the others. The success of this program depends on three things: the patient's attitude toward the program, the level of illness in the body, and their commitment toward overall health. In my experience, this program works to the degree that the patient makes the choice to work within its guidelines."

He agreed to do his best if I promised to do mine. With that, he gave me a reassuring smile and closed my file. As we stood to leave, I had a powerful epiphany—it was I who was ultimately responsible for my health. He was merely a part of my support team, an integral part to be sure, but really, just a part.

Too often we expect doctors to make us well when, in fact, *we* are the only ones capable of doing that. The body will gravitate toward healing when given the proper environment. This was what Dr. Gonzalez was providing me. The rest was in my hands.

As he walked us out, a warm feeling flooded my body and I knew he felt it too. In the hours we'd spent together, a bond between doctor and patient had formed. It filled me with a renewed sense of hope. As we left his office, he suggested we go out and celebrate by eating anything I wanted because once I reached home, all that was going to change. With that he gave us a wink and we left.

We walked down the street feeling the worst of it was over. An incredible burden had been lifted from our shoulders. So much had happened in the past two years that we'd hardly had a chance to be newlyweds. Now, knowing there was hope for a future together, we could let loose and enjoy the rest of our trip. We decided to make this meal a celebration of my renewed health and our life together.

Searching for the perfect place to eat, I noted we were both more relaxed than we had been in over a year. That alone was cause for celebration. After a wonderful meal, we made our way back to the hotel for a satisfying night's sleep and some cuddling, something we hadn't done in a very long time.

The next day we flew back to Los Angeles, feeling confident I was finally in charge of my health. I had learned so much about myself over the past months. I felt excited about the next phase of my journey, sure I was finally on the right track. I was being given a second chance and I was determined to make the most of it. For I knew in my heart of hearts, I might not get another.

15

Cancer Becomes My Teacher

Once home, with no place to run, the reality of my situation hit me full force. Where to begin? First, I needed to eliminate everything in my kitchen cupboards and refrigerator that was remotely good or tasty. I knew the temptation would be too much. For the foreseeable future only fresh, organic, unprocessed food was allowed. For Scott, this meant eating most of his meals out of the house or being subjected to my diet.

We hadn't specifically discussed his changing his eating habits but he had intimated on the trip home it wouldn't hurt him to pay better attention to his own diet. I certainly didn't expect him to adhere to my program but since I was already feeling deprived before I had even begun, I knew it would be a big help to me.

In a tremendous show of support he agreed to not bring home cookies, cake, pie or other pastries. I knew what a sacrifice that was for him and with my birthday coming up, passing up the obligatory cake was going to be a challenge for both of us.

It wasn't long before our tiny kitchen and living room were transformed into a health food store. Pills, formulas for cleansing, organic produce, and bags of organic coffee were everywhere. Looking at all the things I needed to take, the foods I needed to eat and the new routines I would have to perform, it suddenly seemed overwhelming.

And lest you think Dr. Gonzalez was letting me have coffee, that's not exactly what the coffee was for. One of the demands of the program was doing coffee enemas three times a day. Now, I don't know about you but in my circle of negative childhood memories, enemas are right up at the top of the list!

Dr. Gonzalez had explained that cancerous tumors give off heavy amounts of toxicity that poison the body. Couple that with the everyday toxins the body deals with and it's not surprising our systems become overloaded. According to Dr. Gonzalez the cleaner the body, the easier it is to bring it back into balance and enemas were a way to flush out toxins. For better or worse, they were about to become a part of my life.

Eager to get comfortable with my new life, I flopped down on the floor and began putting together packets of pills in plastic bags. It took me two hours to do one week's worth of pills. I was beginning to understand what Dr. Gonzalez meant by "being committed to getting healthy." I could see this was going to require herculean discipline just to put together the pills each week, much less clean, peel, and juice all the raw organic vegetables I was required to eat each day.

My particular plan included taking close to one hundred forty pills—vitamins, herbs, minerals, and pancreatic enzymes—on a very strict schedule. This required my rising by a certain time each morning so I could complete taking my pills by nine o'clock each night. In addition, I needed to set my alarm for three o'clock every morning to take my pancreatic enzymes. This schedule was fifteen days on and five days off. A schedule that in and of itself was exhausting. At first I looked forward to the five days off until I realized they were more arduous than the fifteen days of pills.

During the five-day cycle I was required to do specific cleansing routines. The first was a liver flush. This ghastly purge consisted of drinking eight glasses of organic apple juice and phosphoric acid throughout the day, in addition to the other food and juicing. On the fifth day, when I finished my last glass of juice, I was to take a tablespoon of Epsom salts mixed with half a glass of warm distilled water both before and after dinner. And instead of my regular evening meal, I was to drink as much as I could of a liquid shake that consisted of raw whipping cream and organic berries. Then, a half hour before bedtime I had to drink a quarter cup of organic extra virgin olive oil. Upon retiring I was to lie on my right side for thirty minutes.

The Epsom salts alone were more horrible than anything I had ever tasted. Drinking olive oil was no picnic either. The phosphoric acid in the apple juice softens and dissolves gallstones in the gall bladder, allowing easy passage of the soft, shrunken stones. The cream and olive oil cause a strong contraction of the gall bladder and liver, forcing out stored waste and bile. The liver flush to improve liver function also helped to lower the cholesterol levels in the body.

As I had suspected, the routine was grueling. Believe me, nothing short of knowing my life was at stake could have kept me committed to this program. I was fully aware these harsh treatments were drastic measures for a drastic disease.

The day after my first five-day cleanse I could hardly move. Every fiber of my being ached. I was so alarmed at how I felt that I called Dr. Gonzalez's office in a panic, but his nurse assured me my body was reacting exactly the way it was supposed to. She called it a "healing crisis" and told me I would go through several over the next year. *God, please no*! I thought. *A year of this?* Maybe I didn't have to worry about the cancer killing me—this program would!

And as if that five-day cleanse wasn't enough, there were two additional five-day periods each month that required other specific cleansing routines. One was called the "clean sweep." This consisted of a mixture of finely ground psyllium seeds and clay three times a day for a total of fifteen doses. Upon finishing the fifteen doses, I was to eat plain nonfat yogurt two to three times a day for the next five days to replenish my bacterial flora. The swollen mass of psyllium gradually works its way through the small and large intestines of the body filling every nook and cranny while forcing out all manner of stored waste that would not otherwise be excreted. These wastes can accumulate over a period of many years and seriously interfere with the absorption of nutrients. The clean sweep is also the most effective way of removing abnormal bacteria and other organisms from the gut that often take hold after antibiotic use.

Last, but by no means least, the final cleansing routine was called "the purge." Dr. Gonzalez considered the purge, accomplished while fasting, one of the most important detoxification routines for cancer patients. It puts the body at rest and aids in the rapid removal of metabolic waste. In addition, it pushes the body into an alkaline state in which repair and rebuilding of damaged tissue occurs rapidly.

The purge requires juicing twelve organic oranges, six organic grapefruits, and six organic lemons into half a gallon of distilled water. Upon rising in the morning, I drank one tablespoon of Epsom salt dissolved in half a glass of distilled water. A half hour later I repeated that dose and then again a half hour after that for the third time. Approximately two hours after the last dose of Epsom salts I drank a glass of the citrus punch. Subsequently, I was to drink a glass every hour until it was gone. This was repeated on the second day.

It was quickly clear to me this program was not for everyone. To say one must be highly motivated was an understatement. Sticking to the schedule and tolerating the boredom of eating the exact same meal three times a day were highly challenging. I understood why Dr. Gonzalez had said that sometimes the sicker his patients are, the better they do. You don't have to preach motivation to someone who's looking at death's door.

Dr. Gonzalez had warned me that each patient has a different experience with the program. During the detoxification periods there could be a number of different side effects including nausea, body aches, fever and complete exhaustion. At one time or another, I had them all. But most difficult was merely getting through the rigorous day-to-day schedule while feeling so exhausted and achy.

I also understood why Dr. Gonzalez had cut out my exercise routine. There were days I could barely drag myself across our small studio apartment to the kitchen. Thank God Scott had incredible energy and a great constitution. There were many nights when he'd get home from his second job and clean twenty-five pounds of carrots so I wouldn't have to. He was mostly operating on only a couple hours of sleep each night. I felt so fortunate that God had placed this man in my life. I don't know what I would have done without him to help me through this time. I felt incredibly blessed.

At my initial meeting with Dr. Gonzalez he'd told me I would be on my program for a minimum of two years and possibly up to five. However, the way I was feeling I didn't think I would make it six months. Then, just in the nick of time, a curious thing happened.

Having tenaciously adhered to everything that was required, after just a few short weeks I started to experience a clarity I had never known. Physically, I was still having pretty harsh side effects but this mental lucidity was something completely different. This was more like a fog being lifted from my mind, a clear intuition of what it must be like to feel healthy. For the first time, I was beginning to understand that being healthy extended beyond the physical body. Being healthy was also that spiritual part of me that was creative and expressive. By shutting down this part, I had compromised my immune system's ability to operate at its optimum.

I realized I'd been getting warning signs about this disease for years but had been too unconscious to notice. I thought exhaustion, being hit with colds and flus three to four times a year, lack of clarity, and drastic mood swings were normal. Everyone gets sick, I reasoned. But now, armed with more information I became aware that feeling like crap all the time is not normal and should never be reasoned away. I was waking to the fact that the body is always talking to us. Sometimes the conversation is subtle and sometimes, as in my case, the conversation is not so subtle but communication is always happening. It merely requires that we listen. Something inside me was waking up, and although there was still much to learn, I felt in my heart I was on the right track.

As the months wore on there were times when it was difficult for me to integrate my moments of clarity with my reality. That's when I decided it would be helpful to write in a journal. When I was younger I had had a diary but stopped writing in it soon after getting out of school. *I'm too busy to write*, I thought. *Too involved in getting on with my life to spend time on such silly things. Diaries are for kids. I'm an adult with better things to do!* Now, it felt right to begin again. But this time I would make it a sacred act each day to honor my journey and my thoughts.

I would begin with a prayer, asking that my guides be present. Then I would write down my insights, along with my dreams and any messages I received from my "voice." With each passing day I began to see that the insights and messages were helping me regain balance in my life, moving me into a deeper connection with Spirit. It also served as a vehicle for putting my thoughts and feelings in perspective, giving me a tangible way of expressing my fears, anger, pain, and anything else that bubbled up. My goal each day was not to judge what I needed to express. I simply wrote, allowing my feelings to be, which opened me up to a deeper understanding of myself.

Generally I wrote at the end of each day, but often there would be messages in earlier meditations that were so profound I would write them down immediately. At the end of each week, I would read what I had written and reflect on how I was feeling. These messages helped me become aware of ongoing patterns and habits that were not serving me in my quest to regain my health. Adding this practice to my toolbox helped me gain insight, strength, resolve, and an overall sense of wellbeing.

Although I was vigilant with my program, I had a lot of problems with the diet. After six months, I was sick of eating raw, bland, tasteless food and was ready for a change. Dr. Gonzalez did not share my view and continued to stress the importance of the diet he prescribed. I knew he was right but continued to resist by affirming how much I hated the food. I didn't realize my resistance and negative attitude were perpetuating a scenario that had the potential to turn into a real problem.

One morning, as I began my usual negative rant about breakfast, it occurred to me that by thinking negatively about this food that was helping to heal my body, I was sending a message that there was something wrong with it. This came as a revelation and prompted me to explore what needs I had that I associated with the junk food I craved. Furthermore, I contemplated, why would I want to put junk in my body in the first place? I discovered that over the years I had denied my needs and anesthetized my feelings with unhealthy food.

Every time feelings of disappointment came over me, I would grab something sweet to eat. This would distract me from dealing with the issues that prompted my behavior, giving me a false sense of satisfaction. But now it dawned on me that this pattern solved none of my problems. To realize how damaging this behavior was to my overall emotional, psychological, and physical wellbeing was a huge discovery. What I finally came to appreciate was that I needed to care for myself by not only feeding myself nourishing food but also by giving myself what I needed emotionally. I realized I had a choice to either treat this program and what I was learning as a gift or stay in resistance, threatening the success of my healing.

Exploring this further I began to see that a part of me resisted things that were good for me both physically and emotionally because I didn't love myself. Translated, this meant I didn't want to be healthy. This was a powerful breakthrough. Without the funds for a therapist, practicing meditation, journaling, and prayer had all come together to help me seek higher guidance, a critical component to my ultimate healing.

During this time I also found myself tremendously grateful for everything that had come into my life to support my healing. It struck me as dichotomous that now during one of the most challenging times of my life, instead of asking for things, I was thanking God for everything, including the cancer. This was not a conscious plan or strategy, but simply my mind flowing naturally in that direction. I noticed being grateful made me feel better, while praying out of lack made me feel I was missing something. I would learn later I was actually tapping into a Universal Truth—wherever you focus your gratitude, you create more of that for which you are grateful.

A simple thing like reframing my attitude about deserving good health along with embracing a more positive approach toward my food program started a chain reaction. In meditation and prayer I found myself rethinking and questioning everything I knew about myself in order to change who I had been to become the "I am" of my highest nature.

The cancer was literally and figuratively killing my old self. Because of my illness, I was now on a program that was rearranging my cellular structure and leading me into a deeper connection with the God of all. My survival depended on my letting go of old patterns that had opened the possibility for cancer to emerge and instead embrace health on all levels of mind, body, and spirit. The cancer had come as a messenger to let me know if I didn't change, I was going to die.

A shift from perceiving the cancer as an enemy out to kill me, to a messenger that was in my life to help me change, was profound. Without changing anything but my perception, I turned the cancer into a helpful messenger, a gift. As a result of this disease I was becoming more truthful, more aware, more at peace, and more confident. I could now see my life as a progression, a growth curve along which cancer was one of the mileposts. Having cancer no longer made me a victim but was instead a wake-up call to my divinity.

As more insights dawned, I was given strength and hope to continue my healing program, allowing me to embrace life in a way I never had before. I became willing to change my perceptions about my present and my past. I was able to see the experiences and people I had judged so negatively in my life through different eyes, eyes that perceived them from a place of compassion and grace. And I was finally accepting one of the greatest gifts of all: a heart that was coming alive to the power of forgiveness.

As I continued asking for guidance to explore these areas, I practiced looking at the events in my life from a higher perspective, a perspective that could see them as serving me on my path to greater awareness. This took a while to get used to, because frankly, this had not been a very operable concept to me. But with each new revelation, I became so intrigued and grateful for the changes taking place in me that I decided to seek out more books on self-help and spiritual awareness. My appetite to know and understand these new concepts was insatiable.

It became more and more clear to me I needed to take responsibility for all the circumstances in my life, including my health. I thought, *If one has the ability to create a disease through bad habits, poor diet, and negative thinking, then one also has the potential power to create health by changing that dynamic within.*

I was finally seeing a glimpse of a bigger picture. When I walked away from chemotherapy, I embarked on a path to a new way of thinking and being. Because I refused the quick fix, I was guided to seek answers from inside. I was forced to go on an inner exploration that challenged me to let go of my resistance and trust what was showing up in my life. Each time I did, I was guided forward and the result was a stronger, more confident me.

Using this approach to wellness, I was able to create a new vision of healing. It opened me up to receive divine intervention, something that a few years before I would have labeled hogwash. Now, I was operating on the advice of an internal voice that was guiding me toward newfound wisdom.

While the books I read were a tremendous help, there was also a highway of information that seemed to show up magically, as if out of nowhere. And as Divine Order would have it, right when I needed it. For the first time in my life, I was discovering the "I am" at the core of me. And from somewhere deep inside, I knew it was this new me that would save my life.

In the days and weeks that followed, my understanding of these concepts grew and deepened, becoming a powerful tool I used in my healing. Feeling more in charge of my life, I made the conscious decision to stop resisting any part of my program. I would use what I was learning as a working model for getting well, all the while keeping in mind that the cancer had indeed, become my teacher.

16

The Pupil Learns

Feeling that life was finally moving in a forward direction, I gratefully embraced the changes. That is, all but the changes in my marriage. With each of us focused on our separate roles, Scott and I were spending less and less time together. Whenever the subject of our relationship did come up, we rationalized our circumstances. We'd talk about my disease or our money concerns, convincing ourselves we were working on our marriage, but the truth of the matter was, neither of us could face what was happening. With all the growth taking place in my own being, it became increasingly more difficult for me to deal with what was becoming of us.

Scott had come to resent my condition and the sacrifices he'd made, and although his attitude hurt me, I understood why he felt that way. As far as our relationship was concerned, his sacrifices and my guilt about them were a deadly combination. Unable to talk about how we felt, our relationship became increasingly more distant.

And when it came to sexual intimacy, well, let's just say, it didn't. Sex was not on my radar. I literally had no energy for it. All my focus was on healing. I didn't feel sexy. The loss of my breasts, along with the prominent scars from my surgeries made me feel less than desirable. And though I wanted to share this with Scott, I wasn't able to. In addition to the shame I felt, I also felt like he was unavailable. As things continued to fester between us, we promised each other that as soon as our circumstances and my health changed for the better, we would recommit to our marriage.

In spite of the sadness and confusion I felt about what was happening with Scott, I was feeling stronger and more optimistic about my health with each passing week. Much to my relief, the reports I was getting from Dr. Gonzalez corroborated this. And though I knew it was an important part of my healing to deal with negative feelings that bubbled up, I figured I could deal with them once I got back on my feet.

I was finally experiencing a new and welcome phenomenon—what it felt like to get healthy. Previously when I reported to my doctors that I didn't feel well, they told me my tests were normal and I was fine. But in reality, the opposite was true. My tests may have appeared normal, but my body was fighting cancer and no one had diagnosed it.

One of the things I loved about my program was the total participation I had in my own healing. Dr. Gonzalez confirmed what I had felt all along, that my body did know what was going on. He welcomed my input and always compared what I was experiencing against his test results. Consequently, I felt not only empowered but looked forward to getting my updates every three months.

Through the process there were constant adjustments in the supplements to accommodate my progress. Dr. Gonzalez was able to determine where my body chemistry was out of balance and how my immune system was responding. If a report showed a deficiency in a particular mineral, he would slowly increase the dose of that mineral supplement.

I became so sensitive to the messages my body was sending that I was able to head off more serious problems by correcting imbalances before they became too great. I was learning to read my body not only on a physical level but opening up on all levels, emotionally, mentally and spiritually. And though I followed my program religiously, there was a point where my physical stamina began to wane and I knew I was seriously out of balance.

However, having realized the power of listening to my body I was able to systematically eliminate certain supplements I felt were no longer agreeing with me. I knew I was taking a chance that I not only could be wrong but also could be cut from the program. Dr. Gonzalez had made it abundantly clear that I was to follow his instruction without question or risk being dropped as a patient. But no longer willing to ignore my body's signals, I carried on with my self-assessment, adjusting my supplements as I saw fit, eager to see what my next set of tests would reveal.

When my next report arrived, it verified what my intuition and body had told me. Going through my report with Dr. Gonzalez, he instructed me to stop taking some of the same supplements I had already discontinued. It was the proof I needed that there was a divine intelligence working through my body. All that was required was that I remain open to the communication I was receiving and act accordingly. It took a long time for me to accept that the process of healing is not an experience separate from us but rather a part of life as a whole.

About two and a half years into the program, I was doing so well I began to go on autopilot. With my quarterly hair analysis report coming up, I was fully expecting a positive result. However, this time was different. This time the report, performed to determine cancer rate, reflected a significant rise in mine. Dr. Gonzalez was so concerned about it he immediately called to find out what was going on.

"Brenda," he inquired, "are you following instructions without deviation?"

"Absolutely!" I reported.

"Everything?" he quizzed. "All supplements? Cleansing?"

"Yes, yes. Everything!"

"And your diet?"

"To the letter!"

"What is going on in your life? Emotionally. What is up?" he queried.

My stomach locked and my mind drew a blank. Here it was. The part of the equation I had to face if I was ever going to get well. I knew I had to go deeper within and deal with the life issues I had so successfully avoided.

News that my cancer rate was on the rise shook me to the core. And though I knew what needed to happen, what I didn't know was how to facilitate it. So, after I hung up the phone, I did the only thing I could think of. I got down on my knees and I prayed. I prayed for guidance. I prayed for a way to release the guilt that was eating away at me. I asked to be shown the lessons I needed to learn so I could forgive myself. So I could release Scott from the resentment I felt.

Over the months I'd been on the program I had become totally and completely dependent on Scott. He was overworked and rapidly wearing down from the stress. To further complicate things, Hollywood was in the middle of an actors' strike, significantly reducing the amount of production work available. This put even more stress on our finances and with it the possibility I might not be able to remain on my program. And while I was grateful for all he had done, I knew we both had some healing to do around our circumstances.

So I prayed. I prayed with faith in my heart that the answers I needed would come to me when I was ready to receive them. I prayed knowing that my prayers would be answered. And then I did my best to let go and let God.

What I didn't yet understand was that most of the underlying issues that continued to limit me had layers. Layers that would surface again and again until I finally resolved the core beliefs at the root of my misperceptions. I hadn't yet discovered that until we heal our negative core beliefs, we continue to encounter the same problems over and over until they are resolved. They may appear to us in a different way. They may even be disguised in such a way that we believe them to be a totally different issue. But when we look honestly, we see that they are, at the core, the same.

One of my core beliefs had always been that I am not enough. In fact, I believe that is a universal core belief. It plays itself out in numerous ways but one of my ways was around money—I never had enough. So to work out that part of my core belief, I attracted a mate who had the same issue. Not surprisingly, our financial situation was always in jeopardy.

While I was working on changing my "I am not enough" paradigm, the strike in Hollywood was going into its third month. It was clear we had to do something. Since the only other place for Scott to make money was Seattle where he was a licensed and established builder, we began to explore the idea of moving back.

Symbolically, this was a blow to both of us—it meant accepting defeat, going backwards, admitting that everyone was right, we couldn't make it in Hollywood. But we felt we had no choice. We were in dire straits and had to take action soon. If we didn't create an income source, we would find ourselves without the means to live.

In my consult with Dr. Gonzalez, he assured me it was my emotional state and nothing more that was having an adverse effect on my health. The stress I was holding in my body was putting stress on my immune system and adversely affecting my healing process. And though we needed to make something happen immediately to change our living circumstances, I knew it was even more important that I explore my feelings around my current situation and heal any toxic underlying beliefs once and for all.

One of the big revelations for me during this time was that I was putting too much emphasis on my program. I had disproportionately turned it into some kind of wonder drug not realizing it was only one of the factors contributing to my healing. My job was to remain as vigilant in my spiritual practices as I was with my diet and supplements. I needed to make sure I didn't lose sight of the interconnectivity of my emotional healing, my physical wellbeing, and my spiritual centeredness.

This was a constant challenge because my habit of denying and repressing my feelings was so familiar. When stressful events appeared in my life, my pattern was to shut down my heart, protecting myself from pain. It was much easier to intellectualize my problems into submission. When that didn't work, I would drink too much or eat too much sugar or spend money I didn't have. I did anything and everything I could to distract myself from facing my problems.

I unwittingly encouraged my mind to offer up one solution after another without ever getting to the core beliefs that sponsored the problems in the first place. I was conditioned to believe the mind knows how to solve problems. But the mind offers only temporary fixes. Having cancer taught me the hard way that healing negative, limiting beliefs, misperceptions, and denied emotions is the most important thing we can do if we want health and wellbeing in our lives. This is authentic healing . . . mind, body and spirit coming into harmony to create optimum health.

After many months of grueling self-examination, I began to see that at the root of "I am not enough" were three distinct elements: fear, judgment and resistance. All my pain and suffering were the consequence of these. I was learning that what I feared, I also resisted or judged. I became aware that living this way created disease in my body.

I began to take notice of how fear, judgment and resistance affected me. I began to consciously make different choices than I had in the past and miraculously, amazing things showed up in my life to support me. Friends I could depend on began to appear. Some of these friends were new, and some were friends I hadn't seen or talked to in months or years. People I had never met connected with me, many of them going through exactly what I was going through. They recommended books and articles in magazines that helped me tremendously. Guidance was showing up in unexpected ways, adding to the feeling that there was more to this than met the eye. I began to feel safe and protected and became a believer of the adage, "When the student is ready, the teacher appears."

I thought back to the day I'd sat in Dr. Gonzalez's office and made the commitment to do his program. On that day I also made a commitment to discover myself on a deeper level. My desire to be healthy was a pledge to be healthy in all ways, not just the physical. By making this vow I was giving myself permission to finally get beyond my disease and release myself from bondage.

Verbalizing the commitment was one thing; doing something about it was something else. I knew it would take tremendous discipline, something that had been lacking in my life. In fact, before I got sick I didn't know the meaning of discipline. But the universe in its wisdom helped me create a situation via my illness where my choice became get disciplined or die. At that point, the choice seemed pretty clear.

But how would I find that within myself? There was no one standing over my shoulder watching my every move, no one giving me answers or telling me what to do. I was alone every day, left to my own devices. Left to go crazy or go within. I found the process incredibly difficult. I was social and outgoing. How could I shut that down enough to be still and listen?

When I first began the practice of going within, I would go into my closet, sit in the corner where it was completely dark and try to meditate. When that didn't work, I tried taking a candle into the closet where I would stare at it, willing my mind to be still. That only gave me something else to worry about. What if I set my clothes on fire and burned the place down? *I know, I'll take a clock in the closet and the ticking will soothe me.* You guessed it. Not soothing, just loud and distracting.

Day after day my frustration increased as I emerged from my closet furious that I couldn't be still. How do people shut out the chatter and get in touch with Spirit? What was I doing wrong? And there it was. The answer to my question was in the question. My goal had been to do it right. I needed to control the situation, to make something happen. I was screaming at Spirit, "Give me peace and give it to me *now!*" Sure that I was missing something, I reasoned there must be another way.

One day I made the decision to just be present without needing any particular outcome. In other words, I surrendered to the process. I began to connect with my breath and before I knew it, found myself in an altered state. Thirty minutes passed without my even realizing it. The answer was so simple. There it was again: simple, but not easy!

I uncovered a valuable insight that day. My need to be in control coupled with my attachment to results was hindering me in countless ways. Once I let go and let God, I entered my space, both literally and metaphorically, allowing a meditative state to evolve naturally. I was able to sit comfortably, putting my attention on my breathing. I would follow my breath in and out until there was no separation between my breathing and my being. And though my mind would occasionally wander, I didn't try to control it. I simply put my attention back on my breath. When I stopped trying to get answers, a wealth of information came to me through my inner voice.

Soon my meditative practice became second nature and I looked forward to the daily time alone with myself. There were certain questions I wanted answered and I started to use my practice as the path to find them. Each day before beginning, I would take a moment to jot down the questions in my journal. Then during my meditation, when I felt inspired, I would ask. As my connection to Spirit grew, I became more courageous, asking some pretty tough ones.

I asked the cancer what it represented in my life. An amazing vision began to take shape: a small white box wrapped with blue velvet ribbon was presented to me. Receiving it, I examined it carefully. I slowly untied the bow, lifting the top off the box. The word CANCER in big, bold letters sprang directly out of the box as if the evils from Pandora's box had been unleashed. Shocked and scared, I jolted out of my meditative state, immobilized, unable to stop shaking. Uncontrollable tears ran down my face as my mind started to spin a story about what had happened.

My mind, fighting for the upper hand, began telling me the cancer was not going away as I thought it was. My mind assured me that not only was I not healing, I was going to die. It went on to invalidate everything I was doing and learning. In a powerful show of force, my mind was letting me know it was in control. It not only had me convinced I was headed down a path of no return, but it recruited my fear and anxiety for support.

By the time Scott got home that evening, I was a mess. And for all we had been through, he listened as he always did and tried to comfort me.

"Brenda," he said gently, "I'd like to propose that maybe there's something more to this than you realize. Maybe there is a deeper meaning to what you heard."

I didn't trust myself to speak but looked off as if the answer was in the candle burning on the table.

"Brenda?" he said, forcing me to look in his eyes. "Can you hear me?"

"Yes," I muttered.

"Why don't you try going back into meditation and ask for the true meaning of your vision?" he suggested.

"Maybe. I don't know," I offered lamely, my fear so deep I couldn't see anything else.

"Brenda," Scott coaxed. "Try it. What have you got to lose?"

Well, that was true. What *did* I have to lose?

"I'll think about it."

"Promise?"

"Promise."

A couple weeks later, after being depressed and on edge, I was desperate. I decided it was time to face my fear. I needed to find out exactly what the cancer vision meant. Girding myself, I began the process of going inside. I asked to be shown the meaning of my vision. Nothing came. As the days passed and I tried harder to get an answer, I became frustrated and angry.

Then one morning, following a night of concentrated prayer, I awoke feeling invigorated and positive, something I hadn't felt for a long time. It helped ease me into meditation with a light heart and a willingness to let go of the need to get the answer. As soon as I surrendered, the answer came to me in the form of a beautiful voice. It told me my cancer was a gift and as I stayed with this feeling, it informed me the cancer was there as a catalyst in my life. It had come to propel me toward my spiritual growth, assisting me in transforming my negativity into life-affirming perspectives and beliefs.

Coming out of meditation, I realized I had been allowing my mind to control me. I had let fear dominate my thoughts and consequently my mind had misinterpreted the vision. It was only when I let go and trusted the Universe, when I released the need for a specific outcome and simply connected with Spirit that I was able to hear my inner knowing. This knowing was what was real. My thoughts were just that. Thoughts! And thoughts possess only whatever meaning we assign them. They can disguise themselves as the truth, but they are not.

It was a powerful demonstration of how fear that roots in the mind can lead to erroneous conclusions. Never again would I reach for guidance with my fear-filled mind. Instead, my new goal was to trust the information from Spirit, knowing we get what we are ready to receive and never more than we can handle.

As I looked back to that day lying on the bathroom floor anguishing over losing my second breast, I realized how perfect it had been. Spirit knows how to get our attention and always, though many times it doesn't feel that way, with love. Having cancer and losing my breasts, while painful, was the perfect lesson for me. I needed that kind of a jolt.

I had been totally invested in how I looked. I was invested in being right, being in control. Most importantly, I was determined to do and be something that was not in accordance with my soul's destiny. Certainly Spirit could have used something else to awaken me, but the loss of my breasts, along with the surrender this experience required of me, showed me how powerful I am. It opened the way for me to choose the highest and best for me, something I hadn't been able to do previously.

I was finally ready to receive the truth and as a result my healing took a giant step forward. I was discovering that beyond curing this disease, beyond taking responsibility, beyond surrender, the cancer was giving me an opportunity to transform all my negative beliefs and patterns. I now had the opportunity to be all I was meant to be. My long-hidden passion had been ignited clearing the way for my mission to begin.

17

Living in the Present

With some of my most pressing questions answered, my world opened up for more and deeper questions to surface. *Why*, I wondered, *did I need to create something as life-threatening as cancer to wake me up?* At first, no concise answer emerged but soon bits and pieces began to fall into place. In one of the many self-helps books I read during this period, a quote from Anthony Robbins jumped out at me: "People either move forward out of desperation or they move forward out of inspiration." It went on to explain that oftentimes it takes an event that creates desperation for people to be humbled enough to surrender the ego mind to the higher self. That was certainly true for me. Nothing before my cancer had threatened me enough to ask, *Who am I?* or *Why am I here?*

Before the cancer, I was consumed by fearful thoughts of self-pity and feelings of lack. I processed everything in my life from a foundation of negativity and looked for what was wrong with me and everyone else. It never occurred to me to look for what was right and wonderful. I blamed everyone and everything for the dismal circumstances of my life. I resisted on every level, completely unaware of the divine present in all things. And of course I had never expressed appreciation for anything. Now, ironically, in spite of the cancer, I was so grateful for all the blessings and insights fueling my experience.

Part of taking responsibility for my life meant accepting the correlation between my fear, my negativity and my cancer. And conversely, if fear and negativity contributed to my cancer, might not love and a positive attitude contribute to my wellbeing? The answer was now so obvious. How could I have not seen it before? So, I chose to change my perceptions about life; I chose to undertake new positive beliefs that supported me in every way.

I noticed one way to stay positive was to stay in the present. The most spiritual among us know this is the ultimate state of awareness. Brooding over or living in the past brings more experiences from the past and plops them squarely in the present. Living in the future induces fear of the unknown. By living in the past and not healing the wounds that bound me I was living in a dis-eased state. Now I was learning it was best to see my past as a teacher, to use it as a tool for understanding myself better and to let these new understandings inform my future, allowing it to unfold naturally.

The body doesn't discern its response to emotions as happening in the past or the future. It only interprets them as happening in the now. The body is always in the present. It is the mind that has a thought that triggers an emotion. And though the mind may know it is considering an event from the past or the future, the body does not make that distinction. It became clear to me that by allowing my mind to constantly dwell on the past and/or future, it stimulated emotional responses that became excess baggage for me in the present.

When I consciously practiced keeping my thoughts moment-centered, I felt empowered. If my thoughts drifted to the past, I didn't resist but instead felt gratitude for knowing the difference. I would acknowledge my past for giving me my present awareness. When I worried about a future event, I would deal with it in a positive way, visualizing exactly what I wanted to happen and seeing myself healthy and vibrant. Then I would return to the present moment and deal with what was directly in front of me.

I was learning to put my thoughts on what I wanted as opposed to what I didn't want. As I continued this practice each day, I gained more inner strength and self-confidence. When my mind would wander, I trained it to go toward things I wanted and felt positive about. With fewer negative judgments about my past or future, I found I wasn't as negative in the present. Living like this helped me feel physically better and spiritually more uplifted. Although this took focus and discipline, the rewards far outweighed the time and energy it took. Living this way started to become automatic and effortless.

Now, that's not to say I had it conquered. It was an absolute necessity to be vigilant in my pursuit of peace. I would review my journal from time to time to see if there were still patterns that stood out.

Not surprisingly, there were. I noticed the underlying theme of martyrdom and self-sabotage playing out over and over in my life, causing me extreme pain and disappointment.

I had spent most of my life nurturing and doing for others, letting my own needs and desires take a back seat. I thought the only way anyone would love and accept me was if I overcompensated for my self-perceived lack. I ignored my own needs and generally suffered as a result. I would often end up resenting the people I martyred myself for, only to punish them later by making them feel guilty for not appreciating me. This emotionally dysfunctional merry-go-round became a vicious cycle in my life, draining me of self-worth and creating toxic relationships.

What I would eventually discover is that the universe serves as a mirror. Everything we think and feel about ourselves is mirrored back to us through our relationships, our behaviors and the circumstances we create. As a martyr, it was easy for me to be the victim who could justifiably blame circumstances, people, or life in general for every negative situation I experienced. Then I could harbor feelings of anger, resentment, guilt and punishment as a payback to those who wronged me.

I was well aware the common denominator fueling all my negative beliefs, patterns and perceptions had been birthed out of some aspect of fear. Tracking this was not difficult since it was where I focused my attention. It was what I thought and talked about. It was the motivating factor of all my actions. I repeatedly used my God-given right to choose and aimed it toward fear instead of where I truly longed to live, surrounded by love.

I was coming to realize if I wanted peace of mind and love as my mainstays, I couldn't continue to hold on to the negative core beliefs that supported my fear. I started to see that my thought patterns played out as my experience and if I wanted a different experience, I needed a different thought pattern. That is when I made the choice to see the gift in everything, regardless of how things might be playing out on the surface.

I realized I needed a ritual to rid myself of the negative layers of misperceptions that had driven my life. Negative thoughts and fear create toxic debris. To release this debris, I would focus on taking several deep breaths while consciously turning my thoughts to peace. Once calm, I would imagine myself in a tunnel, surrounded by white light. I'd gather all my negative feelings, visualize them in various colors, and release them into the light. I would then replace the old toxic feelings with feelings of love, forgiveness, joy, or whatever came to me in the moment. Religiously performing this ritual became a very powerful way for me to cleanse myself of the toxicity I had carried for years.

This simple process of coming to grips with my fear brought me to another level of peace and acceptance as I learned to engage them in a dialog. In this process, I would welcome my fears into my space and ask them why they were there. Almost every time they would tell me they were there to teach me something. Embracing my fears rather than resisting them taught me a very powerful lesson that was about to test me.

One day in the middle of my usual cleansing routine, I noticed a small lump in my groin. Sure the lump must be cancer, my fear level shot through the roof. In a split second all the work I had done dissipated as I felt myself sinking into desperation.

Simultaneously, my mind told me everything I had done to that point had been a waste of time. What a fool I'd been, thinking I was getting better. It was a painful, recurring theme that echoed the vision I'd had about the white box, but at the time I didn't make that connection.

The longer I lay there, the more negative my thoughts became. Soon I was convinced I might as well give up; resign myself to an early death. But something inside urged me to put my hand on the lump. I thought perhaps if I touched it I might find I was possessed of some magical power that would make it disappear.

Moments passed. Then minutes, nothing. Resisting my impulse to allow fear to overtake me, I heard, "Breathe. Breathe in peace." Practice what I had been learning? What a novel idea! I did my best to let my negative thoughts pass through my mind, not holding on to any one destructive possibility. When the fear surfaced I would embrace it, breathe through it, and send love into the swelling.

My first inclination was very negative. I knew this was my ego trying to maintain control. I continued to breathe, allowing my fearful, negative thoughts to come and go while sending love to my body. I asked why my body had produced this lump and what message it was trying to give me.

A few moments passed. I heard, "Your lymph glands are blocked. A build-up of toxins in your system."

What? I thought. *How would I know this?*

And on the heels of that thought, I remembered hearing Dr. Gonzalez explain early on that through the process of healing, cancer cells would break down rapidly and need extra cleansing routines to deal with the toxic waste.

Although I had been dedicated to my detoxifying regimens, it was clear my body was breaking down the cancer cells at a rate it could not handle. I realized what I needed to do was step up my detox procedures. So, over the next three weeks I increased my routines and slowly but surely the lump began to dissipate until it was completely gone. I had fought through the layers of fear and won.

Through this process I learned another valuable lesson: not all fear is negative. There were times during my illness when fear presented itself to me as a warning, capturing my attention so I would take action. Fear is negative only when it runs our lives, paralyzes us, or causes us to do unloving things to others or ourselves. There is no need to demonize fear or make it our enemy.

This experience reminded me that even though I was committed to getting well, I was still finding my way. I was still "in process" and had to accept that life could throw me a curve ball at any time. It gave me the opportunity to stop resisting the natural flow, to continue to trust my inner voice and pay attention to the messages my body was sending.

Here it was again. The message I would encounter repeatedly throughout my program. Getting well is the process, not the end in itself. I needed to be with that process. I needed to invite in every seeming diversion along the way. I needed to adopt the adage, "Life is what happens when you're on your way to your goal." I needed to celebrate the process with all its quirks, engaging every twist and turn no matter what. Knowing that when I stayed in the present, life would unfold in all its perfectly imperfect perfection!

Part Four

The Gift of Healing

18

Loving Myself Back to Health

As I learned to tune into my body in new and powerful ways, my confidence gained momentum. I was excited to move ahead, back to my normal life, or at least begin the process of establishing my new normal. But as I had been reminded repeatedly, the process had many layers.

It was during a meditation that my inner voice spoke once again about forgiveness. It told me there were many people I must forgive if I was going to move forward. The name at the top of the list was mine. I hadn't given much thought to the concept of forgiving myself. What did that mean exactly? And though I didn't have the answer at that moment, I had made the commitment to do what needed to be done to heal. If this was part of it, I was ready.

As far as forgiving others was concerned, I thought if I wasn't spending time thinking about them, then I must have forgiven them. Besides, if I'd expressed my feelings and let them know I was angry, didn't that constitute forgiveness? As I sat with these thoughts, I became curious about the true meaning of forgiveness. I'd never thought to include myself in the process. After all, wasn't it someone else's fault if they'd betrayed and hurt me? But if I was to believe the messages I was receiving, I was obviously missing something. I asked what I needed to do to truly forgive. Knowing the answer would appear when I was ready to receive, I went about my business.

Rarely leaving my apartment, I had nevertheless established a pattern of occasional walks or trips to the market. Mondays, Tuesdays, Wednesdays and Fridays I took leisurely walks, wrote in my journal, read my favorite books, and napped. Thursdays I went shopping for supplies and spent time with friends. Saturdays and Sundays were dedicated to Scott.

Since I rarely varied my routine, I was surprised one Wednesday when I felt the urge to visit my favorite health food store. Standing in the checkout line, an attractive woman noticed the copious amounts of coffee I was purchasing.

"Opening your own Starbucks?"

"Oh," I said, feeling oddly like I'd been caught with my hand in the cookie jar. "I'm on a healing program. I need large amounts of certain foods and coffee for cleansing."

"That makes a little more sense," she said with a smile.

I was immediately drawn to this woman. There was something so authentic about her. I felt an overwhelming connection. During the course of our conversation I shared with her that I was a cancer patient.

"I figured there had to be some explanation. You don't look like the barista type," she said, grinning at me. "I'm a spiritual healer."

"Really?" I said, trying to seem noncommittal.

"I can tell by your head tilt you're a skeptic," she said, still amused.

"No, not really. I don't know that much about it. You know, how effective it is. What do you do?"

"I do energetic bodywork." Walking together out of the store she continued, "I work with many cancer patients so I have some idea of what you're going through."

"What's the process, exactly?"

"The work I do consists of various Eastern techniques that help me assist the flow of energy through the various meridians of the body."

"Uh huh." And though I had countless questions about what she did, that was the most eloquent thing I could think of to say.

She laughed. "It's not as airy-fairy as it may sound. These methods have been practiced for thousands of years and are highly effective. I have seen some amazing miracles." Her eyes lit up and there was an undeniable aura of peace around her.

"How does it work?" I asked, unwilling to let go of any healing potential.

"There's no prerequisites or anything. Really all that's required is to be open and willing to experience whatever comes up."

"Do you deal with emotions or only the physical body?"

"I don't believe it's possible to heal the physical body without healing all the levels and layers of the self."

And there it was, the answer to the sixty-four-thousand-dollar question. As I listened to her speak about her work with such passion, my flesh tingled with excitement. Everything she was saying resonated with the messages I'd been receiving. I needed her services, of that I was sure. I was also sure there was no cash to pay for them.

"I am fascinated by what you do," I said, feeling the glow of her energy. "And as soon as I get some funds together, I'll contact you. Thank you for sharing your passion." And with that I turned to go to my car.

A moment later she caught up with me. "Listen," she said, "let's work together."

"But, I don't have . . ."

"Don't worry about it. That's not the end-all-be-all of life," she said, gently placing her hand on my shoulder. "We'll work it out."

I couldn't believe it. My heart was flowing over with gratitude. How could I doubt the existence of angels when so many had shown up to support me? I graciously accepted and we made an appointment for the next day. On the drive home I reflected on the "coincidences" happening in my life. Time and again the very people or situations I needed showed up. Could it be there was a divine hand guiding my healing journey? I was beginning to believe there was.

Erin arrived at my apartment with her special table and music she would play during the session. She lit incense, positioned me on the table and instructed me to connect with my breath to allow my mind and body to relax.

"Imagine yourself somewhere totally safe and peaceful. You are protected and relaxed in your safe place."

I quickly surrendered to the calm of my visualization and waited for further instruction.

"As you become aware of any noises or smells, let them move through you."

When I was ready, she began to gently touch various parts of my body. Within moments I felt an incredible surge of energy pass through me.

"What are you doing?" I asked, more curious than frightened.

"My guides are sending energy to your meridian points," she shared.

As I continued to breathe and surrender to the peaceful feeling, I walked from my safe place out onto the beach. It was a cloudy day and the breeze off the ocean was warm and gentle. Sitting on the sand I listened to the sound of the waves. It was so real, I could actually see and hear the seagulls flying above me. I could smell the salt water in the air and feel the sand between my toes as the gentle breeze stroked my face. I was completely immersed in my vision, unaware of what she was doing but conscious of a slight tingling sensation moving across my body.

"Brenda," she said, "see in your mind's eye what you want healed."

I focused on forgiveness. I hoped by healing any unacknowledged wounds, it might help heal the cancer. Looking out over the ocean, I noticed a continuous circle of dolphins leaping from the water. They passed gracefully through a large dark cloud on the horizon and then back in. I noticed a small spot of light in the center of the dark cloud. Suddenly, it began to grow larger and brighter. Awed by what I was seeing, an image suddenly emerged from the light. My breath caught in my throat. I knew it immediately—it was the same image of Christ I'd seen in my hospital room the night of Eric's healing. Overcome with emotion I began to weep.

As Christ stood in the middle of the cloud, his arms outstretched, the dolphins passed through his body in a circular motion. Then a light beam began to extend out from Christ's body to the shore beside me.

A second later, one of the people I wanted to forgive appeared and began to walk down the beam of light toward me. As this person came closer, an overwhelming sense of love washed over me and I stood as we embraced. The anger, hostility, and resentment I had felt before did not exist. All that remained was love and gratitude for this person and the lessons they'd imparted to me.

As the session continued, people I had totally forgotten about appeared and the pattern repeated. It was the most incredible experience of my life. Never before had I felt the power of this kind of love or the peace it brought me. When I finally "came back to the room," I was drenched with tears. I realized I had forgiven everyone on my list, plus many more I hadn't even thought of before. I was filled with an incredible feeling of peace and love for myself. By releasing everyone from the bondage my anger had created, I also released myself. There was no longer anything or anyone to forgive. A heavy weight had been lifted from my being. I felt nothing but bliss. I was free.

When I sat up, Erin was standing at my feet. I could see something had happened to her as well.

"Brenda," she started, "I can hardly say . . ." she paused.

"What?" I gently asked.

"The entire room was filled with a beautiful golden light. It was incredibly powerful. I feel I've been healed right along with you."

It pleased me she had also had a similarly powerful experience. I didn't think I would be able to describe what had taken place.

"This kind of deep healing doesn't always happen."

"Why is that?" I inquired.

"People in a surrendered state who are ready to be healed are the ones who receive a lot of movement. Not everyone is ready for it but I can see you are."

I hesitate to use this oft-heard cliché, but this event changed my life. It redefined my healing process, bringing it to a new level. I hadn't been fully aware of the multiple layers of anger, guilt, shame, hostility, and resentment that remained unhealed within me. Through this process with Erin I discovered how important it was to express my anger in the moment, at the time of conflict rather than holding on to it, allowing it to fester in my body. My session had been a miraculous blessing. I was finally able to release a large portion of negative feelings and shame I was sure had a hand in creating illness in my body.

To this day, I know this event propelled my healing forward. It confirmed that forgiveness is essential to heal not only our bodies but enhance our spiritual growth as well. For the first time I was no longer at the mercy of the negative feelings that had held me in bondage for so much of my life. I now felt a depth of wellbeing and inner peace I had never experienced. Once again the interconnectedness of mind, body, spirit cleared the way for me to release the negativity that was feeding my disease. Negativity that left unaddressed would have continued to fester, affecting every area of my life, particularly my health.

I believe this type of peak experience, if we are open to it, is possible for each and every one of us. These encounters can bring to the forefront universal concepts and truths that can serve our growth. I was then, as I am now, incredibly grateful for the opportunity to embrace these concepts and reap the benefits they offer. Benefits that have continued to serve me throughout my life. Benefits that at the time I couldn't fully grasp.

That day I spent with Erin was the last time we saw each other. We didn't exchange phone numbers so I had no way of contacting her. Some time later I inquired at the store if anyone had seen her, but they had not. It was as if she vanished.

I have often reflected on my experience with Erin. I feel as though God sent her to help me along my way. I have believed in angels all my life. After my experience with Erin, I now believe in what I call *earth angels*. I believe they walk among us all the time. All we have to do is be open to experiencing the magic of life and let God do the rest.

This experience inspired me to learn more about my angels, particularly my Guardian Angel. While in meditation and prayer one day, I asked whom my Guardian Angel might be and how I could connect with this spirit. Day after day I asked and asked again, imploring, willing the answer to come. Then one afternoon I decided to stop pleading and let go. That's when the magic began to unfold.

One evening, settling in to my thrice-weekly sea salt and soda baths, I asked about my Guardian Angel. Because I had to do these baths so often, I created a special ritual with soft music and candles all around. In my relaxed and meditative state, I asked to be given a sign or even better, a name. Coming out of meditation without having received anything, I was sure it wasn't time for me to know.

Suddenly, the sound of the candles sputtering caught my attention and I looked to see the flames burning much higher than normal. I began to sense a presence in the bathroom, a presence so enormous it filled the entire space. I was frightened at first but realized my anxiety would stand in the way of experiencing something amazing, so I began to breathe into my fear until it subsided. My connection to spirit renewed, I made another request. I wanted to be told the name of the presence in the room with me. The name Michael popped into my head and I knew it must be the Archangel Michael.

My new library of books included information about angels and Archangels. When I read about the Archangel Michael I felt a connection different than with any other angels I read about. There was something about him that comforted me, giving me the feeling that someone or something was watching over me.

That night, hearing his name made me giddy. I was excited to communicate with him, when suddenly his presence vanished and the flames on the candles returned to normal. The presence was gone. Disappointed at the brevity of our encounter, I nevertheless felt at peace knowing he was with me. Eventually, when the time was right, I knew I would communicate with him.

Inspired by my experience, I put my intention to communicate with Michael in forward motion. I surrendered to the concept of divine timing releasing my notion of how long it should take. And as Spirit would have it, it wasn't long before I became conscious of Michael's presence, producing a feeling of comfort and protection. I became increasingly aware that this presence was growing stronger as I fine-tuned my senses to what his energy felt like. I liken it to exercising a muscle—the more you practice awareness of forces beyond your five senses, the more aware you become of different energies. Soon you can identify which ones are helpful and which are not.

Excited about this new connection, I was nevertheless afraid to share it with others. I knew it was a bit of a stretch and I certainly didn't want anyone to think I was a kook! Thankfully I had Scott who always welcomed my insights with openness and curiosity.

About three weeks after my initial angel encounter, I was invited to meet a lady by the name of Diane. She taught *A Course in Miracles* and was a practitioner of a therapy called rebirthing. I wasn't familiar with rebirthing but was curious. I learned it's a method of re-experiencing your own birth by inducing a trance state through the use of breathing and guided meditation. In this deep meditative state you can recall your own birth experience. You are then guided to re-frame your original experience to remove and heal any trauma or fear that might have occurred during that time.

I asked Spirit if this process would be beneficial to me and received a resounding, "Yes!" After a very powerful conversation with Diane, I decided to try it. Arriving at the class, I met eight women who were all very devoted to their spiritual awakening. Diane placed us in a circle with our heads in the center where we began our breathing. About an hour into the process, just as I was beginning to re-experience my birth, I felt pain in both my ankles and feet. I tried to ignore it and stay focused on my breathing but the pain became so intense I began to hyperventilate. Alerted by my distress, Diane came over and touched my third eye, whispering in my ear that Archangel Michael was at my feet. She told me to give the pain to him. My immediate response was to deny this was possible since I didn't feel his presence. But Diane assured me he was present, waiting for me to give him my pain. Making a conscious choice to let go, I turned the pain over to Michael and it vanished. I was then able to regain my breathing and continue my process.

At the end of the evening I asked Diane how she knew Michael was present. She said the moment I walked through her door she felt his presence hovering over me and he had been by my side all evening. She commented on what a blessing it had been to have him there as he was able to assist all the ladies that night.

That event was another turning point for me. Not only was my communication with Michael reinforced but again I was struck by the divinity of Diane coming into my life with guidance that helped move my healing forward. From that evening on I was in constant communication with Michael and called upon his healing presence to be with me in all things. I would never again doubt the power of the loving forces surrounding me.

19

Letting Go

With the employment picture not getting any better in Los Angeles, both of us were dreading a potential move back to Seattle. But unable to pay our rent and desperate to get something going, the inevitable happened. We set a plan we hoped would get us back on our feet and made the trek back to the Northwest.

Once in Seattle, we put our plan in motion. My first challenge was to figure out what work I could do while maintaining my rigorous healing program. I literally didn't have a clue what that might be. Scott, on the other hand, had connections and expertise in construction and was doing his best to get work in that industry.

My second challenge was our relationship. Things between us had become more tenuous than ever. The disappointment of leaving Los Angeles weighed heavily on us both and our sex life was still missing in action. Our dreams for a life in the entertainment industry had become an abstract concept and as the days passed I felt Scott's anger and resentment grow. I knew he blamed me for all that had happened and because of his attitude I slowly withdrew my energy from our relationship. With our bruised hearts and shattered dreams we carried on with no real idea of what would become of us.

As it turned out, it didn't matter that we didn't know, for the Universe did. A phone call one morning at three o'clock rocked our world. It was Seth, my friend Barbara's husband. He and Barbara had married three weeks prior and we thought they were still on their honeymoon. Half asleep, I listened as Seth sobbed hysterically.

"Barbara. It's Barbara."

"What?" I said, trying to wake from my haze.

"She's in a coma!"

"What?" I repeated, trying to make sense of what he was saying.

"She's dying, a brain tumor. She collapsed while we were honeymooning. I . . . I don't know what to do."

I was numb. How could this have happened? They were at the height of their happiness, their future holding such promise. I couldn't wrap my mind around what he was saying.

As he continued to share the events that led up to this unimaginable crisis, he admitted his real reason for calling.

"Would you come? Would you come to LA, please? As soon as possible?"

"Well, Seth . . ." I hesitated, trying to wrap my mind around his request.

"I know. I know, Brenda. I know what you're going through but you're the only one who can help her."

"Seth, I don't know if . . ."

"Yes, yes, you are," he pleaded. "Please. Please come."

My heart broke for his pain. I knew what I had to do. What I didn't know was that by answering his call for help that night I was about to change the course of our relationship and learn a tough lesson about healing.

Hanging up the phone, I told Scott what had happened. He understood completely my desire to be with Barbara, so we pooled what little cash we had and I flew to LA for a couple of days. Or so I thought.

When I arrived, Barbara was still unconscious. But by the following day her condition changed as she slowly but miraculously emerged from her coma. Believing I would have a positive effect on her condition, Seth, along with Barbara's family, implored me to stay and work with her. Impressed with how well I was doing, they felt I might be able to help her get well. And though my intuition said this was too much responsibility for me to handle, that I should be home tending to my own problems, I agreed to stay. I loved Barbara with all my heart and felt I owed it to her, and in some way to myself, to try. That night I called Scott to give him the details. He agreed I would be good for Barbara, so with his blessing, I decided to stay a while. I didn't know it would be almost four months.

If I'm honest, my decision to stay in LA wasn't only about helping Barbara. Hundreds of miles away from Scott and my own problems, it was a place to hide. So I embraced my mission, hopeful that in my absence, Scott would realize how precious we were to each other.

In my desire to save Barbara, I forgot one of life's most potent rules: heal thyself first. I made the mistake of allowing my ego to drive my need to help her. Instead of creating the opportunity for her to fully engage in her own healing, by encouraging her to turn inward and explore the cause of her disease, I tried to do it *for* her. And by attempting to do that which only she could do for herself, I ended up exhausted and frustrated.

I needed to save the world, a behavior not uncommon for people who have brought themselves back from life-threatening illness. However, what I've learned in the interim is that service can sometimes cross over into caretaking. And instead of empowering those we wish to help, we do exactly the opposite by trying to do the healing for them. For me, healing had been about discovering myself, the most important part of the process. And though self-exploration often brings the beneficial result of a cure, affecting a cure is secondary.

Barbara didn't have that luxury. She did survive a year beyond her original prognosis by following Dr. Gonzalez's program, but her life never really got back on track. She was religious about following the protocols no matter how hard they became for her but when her tumor returned with a vengeance, what little quality of life she had disappeared.

Everyone was in shock at the news, not sure what to think. Barbara was the only one who initially took it well, although that didn't last. Within a few weeks of the tumor returning, her optimism was replaced by anger. She felt all the routines she had struggled through were a waste of time. Life had dealt her an unfair blow.

Soon after, her family's anger began to surface and I was their target. In my heart, I knew each of us had done all we could for Barbara, but I felt guilty because I wished I could have done more. In the end, it became very difficult to be around her. I dealt with my guilt by justifying that, although Dr. Gonzalez's program didn't keep the tumor from returning, she did live a year longer than anyone had expected— and that year was better than none.

During that year I returned to Seattle trying to keep my relationship intact, but ultimately had to admit we were growing farther and farther apart. Scott was having trouble finding steady work in construction and continued to pursue contacts in the movie industry. His persistence paid off when he was offered a job on the movie *Terminator* and we elatedly returned to LA.

Meanwhile, Barbara's health continued to decline. Three months later as I sat by her side for the last time, stroking her hair, despairing over not being able save her, I watched her drift in and out of consciousness. Seth told me she probably wouldn't recognize me but I wanted more than anything to connect with her one last time and tell her how much I loved her.

After sitting with her for over an hour, I decided to say my good-byes, when she unexpectedly opened her eyes, sat up and said, "Brenda, I'm so glad you're here. I want you to know how much you have helped me and how much I love you." Then, just as quickly as she was up, she lay back on her pillow and drifted away before I could say a word.

I grieved her loss for weeks. When I was able to gather my thoughts I reflected on our experience, realizing the powerful lesson she taught me. There are times a body will die no matter what a person does. Sometimes that is the form that healing takes. It was a painful realization. But the gift she imparted was the knowledge that she would live on forever not only in my heart, but also in the hearts of countless others.

I cannot heal or save anyone but myself. No one can. I can, however, be of service by sharing my experience. I've learned it's important not to expect people to have the same experiences and results I had. All I can do is demonstrate that higher possibilities exist in all situations. Ultimately one must decide alone how to experience that process.

Throughout this ordeal, Scott and I had hung on. But now that Barbara was gone and there was nothing to distract us, we could no longer hide from our issues. There was healing to be done between us and I had to stop running from what we had become.

We had been married eight years. Scott's courage, strength and dedication to my wellness went beyond anything I had the right to expect. He was truly an angel in my life. But the consequences of my illness, along with the time spent apart, changed the dynamics of our relationship dramatically. There was no putting our marriage back together. We had moved too far from our foundation to ever be able to repair the cracks.

My heart was broken but my resolve was clear. I was committed to learning the lessons our relationship offered and treasuring those lessons as the gifts they were. The only other choice would have been to spiral down, to allow the hardship and pain endured to become more important than the love shared or the lessons learned. For me the choice was easy. I would honor the years spent together and all we had been through, knowing it would take time to heal my heart.

The intensity of my relationship with Scott taught me about mirroring. As we move through life, we attract and mirror what's happening inside ourselves, making it possible to heal those wounded parts that attract other wounded souls. It's what makes our partners, family, and close friends some of our greatest teachers.

It can help us uncover repressed feelings that live in our subconscious. When we become aware of those feelings, we have the opportunity to heal the misguided perceptions that live beneath them. So often we become angry toward the person who reflected those wounds back to us, not understanding we are the ones who projected these feelings and perceptions in the first place. When we awaken to our role in the process, we can begin to heal our hurt.

Mirroring not only reflects things we need to heal but also reflects the beauty we are as well. The beauty we see in others and the world is the very beauty that lives within. The more we embrace our inner beauty, the more beauty will be reflected back.

I can see now it was no accident that Scott and I were drawn to each other. Having had similar experiences with a dysfunctional family, he mirrored the anger, hostility, shame, and frustration I had carried for years. Because of my disease and what I had learned about mirroring from "A Course in Miracles," I had the time to work on my issues. Overwhelmed, working day and night, Scott did not. He took on that responsibility, pushing his pain and frustration aside. Instead of being able to turn inward for healing and support, he had to put all his energy into our survival.

The dynamic created by my illness didn't allow him to unburden himself. I was aware he didn't want to add to my stress and although I asked him many times if he needed to talk, his response was always the same, "I'm fine." Some might consider him a martyr, others a hero, but whatever side you fall on, the result was a huge amount of armor around his heart. Perhaps he was afraid if he allowed himself to feel too much, he would completely fall apart and be unable to take care of me. Whatever his reasons, the fallout was part and parcel of the debris that remained after we finished our dance through my illness.

I had become stronger and healthier, while Scott became more and more withdrawn. The irony of the effect my illness had on each of us was not lost on me. While I was growing into myself in profound ways, Scott was more angry and resentful than ever. The road we'd traveled together had taken its toll.

After a year or so back in LA, Scott once again immersed himself in the movie industry. He would spend countless weeks and months away from home on location. As the divide between us became more and more defined, we decided to part ways.

Bearing witness to his anger broke my heart. The man I loved and adored more than anything had become a stranger to me. I felt helpless knowing there was nothing I could do to change that. Eventually, Scott sought therapy and I worked on getting back to the lessons I needed to learn to put my life back together.

Being thousands of miles from our families, we decided that for the time being, we would keep our separation to ourselves. We didn't need input from family members who might feel the need to make us wrong for splitting up or for any of the decisions we made during our marriage. We both felt there was no right or wrong, no one person to blame. We knew things happened for a reason and believed good came out of every situation, no matter what appeared to be unfolding. In the end, the love and bond we had from the beginning was still there. It had merely changed as we had changed. We made the decision to honor each other's separate paths to healing. We knew if we were able to make room for the breakup, to appreciate the lessons inherent in its wake, we would each reach new levels of understanding. We owed each other at least that.

In the years that followed, friends would often ask if I thought we might get back together. Through this experience I came to believe we touch each other's lives for a reason, even if it's only a moment, not a lifetime. I knew the moments in time we had shared were extraordinary. There was no question we would forever be bonded in a deep and inexplicable way. If we were meant to be together, we would. If not, Scott knew I would always support his greatness, as he would mine. The rest I was willing to surrender to the Divine.

20

Moving Into Wellbeing

For me, what crystallized next was the ultimate surrender. Once I was willing to let go of whether I lived or died and instead focus fully on the *process* of healing, I found peace. My orientation to life had previously been to hold on tight, control everything and everyone. It made me feel secure, but security is an illusion. I learned that security isn't an outside circumstance, it's an inside knowing.

Letting go brings up fear. My fear said if I let go of control, my life would be chaos. In addition, my fear informed me I was the one who had to "make things happen." But after years of always needing to be in control and do things myself, I grew fatigued and discouraged. No matter how hard I tried or how much control I exercised, there was no guarantee things would go my way. No assurance that people would do what I expected or wanted them to do.

After sheer exhaustion forced me into it, I started to appreciate the power of letting go and allowing God's help in solving my problems. That's when my life began to flourish. Trying to do everything myself, laboring to keep everyone under control, drained every energy reserve I had. Letting go, trusting in a higher power can transcend the need for control and the belief that you have to do it all yourself. And as difficult as this step is, the result—better health and an overall sense of happiness and wellbeing—is unquestionably worth it.

Another "letting go" lesson for me, one I encounter repeatedly as a result of some of the work I do now, is the ability to let go of loved ones whose time has come to cross over. I have been blessed to network with hundreds of cancer patients who enrich my life beyond words; brave beautiful souls who share precious time with me as they move from this life to the next. Not everyone survives this disease, no matter what healing modality they follow. For some, a true healing may come in the form of transition. It is my belief the experience of cancer or any life-threatening disease can, at times, be the vehicle some will unconsciously choose in order to leave this lifetime.

We each hold the key to our own healing. We cannot heal someone else. And when we attempt to do so, we rob them of their highest possibility, even if the highest result is the body making transition. That is not under our control. We do our loved ones a disservice when we hold them here because of our fear of being alone, of not wanting to experience the pain of losing them, or thinking we will never again share the kind of love we have with that person. Our highest duty is to afford them the support and dignity they need to leave with grace, while at the same time holding this truth—all life is eternal.

I believe each individual spirit moves into infinity at the time of death. The only true death is that of the body, since our spirit is eternal. Keeping this in mind can make it easier to let go and bless those whose time has come. It can also be a comfort for us as we deal with our own grief and sense of loss.

There are many things I learned through my cancer experience, but right at the top of the list is that healing isn't exclusively a physical tenet. We must address our emotional and spiritual bankruptcy as well. Once we come to terms with those wounded places within, our healing can move toward completion. We are free to carry on.

Sometimes there will be no perceptible healing before a person crosses over. That is what I witnessed with my father. But his process was perfect for him. We can't know what another has come here to experience. The best we can do is release judgment while allowing the natural process of life and death to unfold in its own unique way according to God's plan for each individual soul.

People may think it takes someone special to accomplish the kind of healing I did. That is not true. Anyone who is ready to look honestly at her life can do what I did, and more. It simply takes a definitive choice to wake up, to commit to a new way of living. The only requirement is to be willing to allow new possibilities to exist and do the work necessary to move into uncharted territory.

As you know by now, I am a firm believer in miracles and divine intervention. And because I believe in them, I am open to experiencing them. During my healing process I found a great deal of comfort in the book *A Course in Miracles*. It was in that book I first read a definition of miracles that resonated with my beliefs: "Miracles are merely our willingness to shift our perception of what's happening in the moment and trust that whatever is there, is there to assist us in our growth."

I cannot stress enough the importance of trust in this process. During meditation and prayer I learned to put aside my preconceived notions of right and wrong, of what I thought was acceptable to everyone else, so I could learn to trust my own guidance.

Being taught early in childhood that my life had limitations and that being a dreamer was a waste of time was devastating to me. It took me years to finally come to the truth that I am unlimited. That's not to say I don't have times when I doubt this truth. But when I do, I often recall an experience I had during my healing.

It happened during a period when I had reached a plateau in my growth. I seemed to be stuck in a spiritual quagmire. Part of my daily process was to walk. Although I lived in a beautiful area, my walk took me past a barren field whose ground was hard as cement. I was sure nothing could grow in the solid, unyielding clay. But this one particular day walking past the field I was startled to see grass popping up everywhere. "Wow!" I thought. "How did this happen?" I was sure I hadn't seen grass in the field the day before.

As I looked on in awe, green grass growing everywhere, I was moved to ask Spirit how this was possible. Spirit answered, "Grass grows because that's what grass knows to do. Nothing can stop this natural motion." My heart warmed and a smile came over my face. I couldn't help but see the correlation between the grass growing and my own growth.

The grass was demonstrating that no matter what our circumstances may be, our destiny is to grow and evolve, to become all we can be. Nothing, not even illness, can stand in the way of our greatness unless we agree to it, unless we take on as truth the information that naysayers would have us believe. For once we accept these thoughts as our own, we act accordingly, giving power to our supposed limitations. This was a powerful reminder for me. I was extremely grateful to the grass for this gift.

Later, as I reflected on this epiphany, I realized that on some level I had been communing with this piece of land all along. The land responded by teaching me I didn't need to worry about my growth as a spiritual being. Everyone's growth and evolvement, including mine, is guaranteed. Our greatness is assured. This is the destiny available to each and every one of us. All the Universe needed from me was my commitment.

Until I was threatened with cancer, I had never truly committed to anything, much less myself. In fact, before my illness I felt there was no purpose to my life and I deserved the "bum deal" I was getting. The experience of cancer taught me that until I was ready to commit to living my life fully, to loving myself unconditionally, the Universe would not support me in what I wanted. In point of fact, the Universe was mirroring back to me what I felt and believed about myself.

When I was first diagnosed, a friend of mine introduced me to Dr. Carl Simonton's book *Getting Well*. In the book, he proposes that his patients ask their cancer what it wants from them. One day in meditation, curious about what the answer might be, I asked the question. The answer I received was that my cancer wanted me to commit to love.

What? I thought. *Commit to loving my cancer?* The concept terrified me. *If I commit to loving my disease*, I reasoned, *it will surely grow and multiply.*

After several days of spending time with this concept, I began to understand that by loving my cancer, I was actually loving myself. Since the cancer was a part of my experience and my soul had called this experience forth, the cancer was a part of me that I needed to embrace. As long as I battled against it, it would battle against me. I realized by loving myself I was filling the "lack" in my life that, on a certain level, was my cancer, my constant companion.

Shortly after this, in another meditation, I received more clarification on love and cancer. This time the message was: *Love doesn't cause cancer to grow, love transforms everything.* This powerful message impacted me profoundly. I finally understood one of life's supreme truths: *Love is truly the greatest healer of all.*

To believe we have no choice about healing our bodies or to deny we have choice at all is to be the victim to our lives. Playing victim keeps us stuck in the "I am not" game. In that game, we believe we are not good enough, deserving enough, smart enough, rich enough, beautiful enough—the list goes on. To heal this great illusion we must be willing to take risks, choose an entirely new way of thinking and being. Until we embrace the truth of our existence, that we are spiritual beings having a human experience, we remain victims, unable to engage in the rich exploration of all we have the potential to be.

There are no right or wrong choices on this journey. Each choice is made for a reason, even those that bring us pain and discomfort. I like to think of it as *divine orchestration*. Every experience is meant to teach us something, while simultaneously bringing us closer to our spiritual selves. To receive each experience with as much grace as possible is to open the window of opportunity to higher consciousness. God is in everything. That includes all our lessons, no matter how tragic they seem.

When I started on my healing path, I was very excited to share my wisdom with everyone. I thought others would be as excited as I was to embrace it. It was my passion, my mission. But as I would come to learn, it was my ego driving this desire for people to heal their lives. My judgment continued in full force, baffled by those who could not see the merit in their own healing. I still had to learn that by not allowing others to choose and trust their own path, I was, once again, trying to control something that was none of my business. I was doing to others what they had done to me when they criticized me for seeking an alternative way of healing. Now I am able to embrace that each of us is unique. Each of us is guided by the divine orchestration at work through our individual lives.

Today, my goal is to be conscious of my thoughts while I look for two things. One, whatever I judge in another, I also carry within me. Two, whenever I judge anyone or anything, every cell in my body constricts. I ask, "What am I afraid of?" and "What would love do?" Once I've asked these questions, I find my need to judge dissipates and an automatic opening is created for a higher possibility to unfold within me. I open the space within to experience peace and feelings of wellbeing that are expansive and energy-giving. I remind myself that every soul is on a spiritual journey of evolution whether they are aware of it or not. It is not my place to tell anyone how, where, when, why, or even if they should heal.

The process of healing calls on our willingness to shift our perceptions of the people and circumstances in our lives. We must forgive, others *and* ourselves, for the supposed slights we fuel with our fear and insecurity. When we are able to do that on the inside, everything on the outside changes. For this process to work, we must first and foremost be willing to surrender to love. When we do that, we can release any resistance to, or judgment about, that which we perceive opposes us. The movement in our lives created by this process opens the door for true transformation. That is what I did with my cancer. By embracing it as a teacher from whom I could learn instead of an enemy that needed to be attacked and killed, I was able to transform my relationship to my illness, thus making it possible for healing to occur.

We have two choices for our life path: to evolve consciously as a loving and empowered being or evolve unconsciously as a victim living in negativity and fear. When we live unconsciously, our choices are extremely limited. This causes fear, anger, depression and a myriad of other negative feelings that lead to illness and *disease*. Becoming conscious opens us to the awareness that we are unlimited and much larger than our senses realize. But even more importantly, a higher consciousness allows us to be *at ease* with whatever events come to us in life, no matter how difficult those circumstances may appear.

My past is a perfect manifestation of that concept. But today I am living proof that growing in consciousness can reverse that pattern. Our greatest challenge is not overcoming illness and disease but rather transforming our consciousness to create a space where the body/mind/spirit can heal. This is the path to living our highest good.

Over the years I have stayed true to my spiritual practices and myself. As a result, I've continued to grow and evolve my consciousness, which has also resulted in my continued good health. It has been twenty-four years since I was diagnosed with cancer and told the probability of living beyond a year was slim. In those twenty-four years I've continued to appreciate my life and all the lessons I continue to learn with an open heart.

It is my sincere hope that what I learned on my journey will provide a road map for you to start your own healing journey, to begin the process of self-love. May God bless you every step of the way as you come to know and accept yourself as a powerful spiritual being forever loved and appreciated.

Addendum

A Lifelong Guide to Wellness

Having regained my health and moved on with my life, I am often asked how I achieved this milestone. On the heels of that is usually an inquiry about the doctor who "cured" me. I am happy to share Dr. Gonzalez's name but am always quick to explain: Doctors do not cure anyone. Dr. Gonzalez and his program were definitely an important part of my support team but healing is a co-creation that includes the patient, the support team and God.

First and foremost the patient must have a deep desire to heal. Giving power to an outside source, regardless of who or what that source is, renders one powerless to change any existing circumstance. I am always sure to make it clear: there are no quick fixes or magic bullets.

It is also vital to understand: *Life is a journey, not a set of goals to be achieved.* This holds true not only for life in general but also for healing. While holding fast to a vision of restored health is essential, it should not be looked upon as the ultimate goal but rather as part of the experience of rediscovering who we are as spiritual beings. When we understand and embrace this principle, healing is possible.

I'd like to share with you here the touchstones I found most important on my healing journey that you might have a head start on your own path to wellness.

Choosing a Physician

Find a doctor with whom you feel comfortable, one with whom you can communicate, one who honors your feelings, intuition, and the wisdom of the messages coming from your body. Make sure your doctor listens as much as he/she talks. Clarify that you both understand completely what is being asked and shared. Ask as many questions as you feel necessary to understand exactly what is going on. Always remember, it is *your* journey and *your* body.

Ask to speak with other patients who have had similar experiences to yours. Find out what they learned and if they had success. You should be able to ask your doctor anything about your condition and receive an answer that satisfies you. If he/she does not answer your questions openly, honestly and willingly, find a different doctor, one who is not only professional but also compassionate. Make sure your doctor is a specialist in your specific illness. If you have breast cancer, find a breast cancer specialist.

Always get a second opinion, no matter what. Two doctors with your best interests at heart are better than one. Once you have chosen a primary physician, check in with yourself and see how it feels to you. Is this the right match? If the answer is yes, you will be able to follow his/her guidelines without second-guessing yourself. Remember to allow your intuition to be a part of your health equation.

Here are some other things to consider:

1. What is the quality rating of the lab where your blood analysis is being done?
2. Does your doctor know how to rate a lab?
3. Does your doctor welcome and work with practitioners of other modalities?
4. Are phone appointments available and is your doctor available to talk to you personally within a reasonable amount of time?
5. Does your doctor respect your feelings and intuition? Is he/she willing to talk to you about these things?
6. Is counseling available for you and your family, and is it welcomed?
7. Is nutrition part of the program?

Once you have found a doctor and all your questions have been answered satisfactorily, the next consultation you should seek is with yourself. This is probably the most difficult thing to do. It's frightening to be given a diagnosis of a life-threatening illness. Try your best not to panic. It's likely taken some time for your disease to develop. Chances are you have more time than you think to do what needs to be done. Unless you have some immediate issue that needs attention, i.e. bleeding, inability to breathe, etc., or are in acute pain, you have time to tune in to your intuition and body. Then do your best to follow what is being communicated.

I know this can be a tumultuous time and the concept of relaxing can be challenging, but try to calm yourself to the best of your ability. Ask that you be connected to Divine Spirit. Ask only questions that result in yes or no answers. You'll remember I asked if chemotherapy would be good for my body and got a resounding "No!" Consequently, I moved in another direction.

Tools to Help You Deal with Fear

It is my belief that Spirit directs everything. We each are blessed with intuition and the ability to cultivate it. By learning to communicate with Spirit, you are tuning into your intuition. This is my approach to achieving that connection.

First, embrace your fear. It is a natural response to a potentially life-threatening situation. You cannot deny its existence, hoping it will go away. The only way to disperse uncomfortable feelings is to look at them head-on as you surrender to them. Once you stop resisting your fear, the energy around it will naturally dissolve and your fear will lessen. The same process works with pain. Remember, what we resist, persists. When we push against our pain and fear, they gain momentum, pushing back at us with an even greater will to maintain their position.

When diagnosed with a life-threatening illness, fear is often generated by thoughts of death. This is not an unexpected response. What I did to help me face those fears was write in my journal about why I was afraid, allowing all my feelings, thoughts and fears to surface. Through this exercise my anxiety and overwhelm began to dissipate. I began to understand it is only the body that dies. Once I allowed my body to move through those feelings, I was ready to work with my intuition to discover the parts of me that needed to heal.

What so often gets in the way of this is our conditioning. In most instances we have not been taught to communicate with our bodies or our Spirit. We don't know how to give ourselves permission to communicate in this way. Instead, we've been taught to believe that Spirit, or God, is out there in the ethers, that our bodies are not living entities with their own intelligence. Many of us don't believe we can communicate with Spirit without the help of an intermediary such as a priest or guru.

We have also been trained to suppress our symptoms rather than embrace them as a messenger. We abuse our bodies with food, drugs, alcohol, sugar and sometimes, meaningless sex in order not to feel. This way of coping is ingrained in our culture. We don't understand that our symptoms are a reflection of our core conflicts through the collective consciousness. We are all part and parcel of the God intelligence.

If you want to know what's going on in your body, your symptoms are your road map. While doctors are able to tell from your symptoms what your physiological problems are, what you want to know is what is causing the symptoms. Getting to the root of your problems is the only way to have a complete healing. This is where your intuition comes in. Your body has its own wisdom that it communicates to you all the time. We simply have not been trained to speak its language or listen for its needs. And even when we do perceive that our body is trying to signal us, we don't trust what it is trying to say.

My suggestion is to set aside time to connect with your body through Spirit. Take some deep breaths, listen to soothing music, tap into the inherent power of the mind, body, spirit connection. If you already have a practice of meditation or prayer, use those techniques.

Once you connect with your breath, your body will begin to relax. Allow any and all thoughts to come and go. Don't fight them. Allow them to pass through your mind. When you have reached a state of relaxation, tune into your symptoms. In other words, focus your consciousness on your symptoms in the area of the body where the pain or symptoms are physically based. Then, request that the pain and/or symptoms communicate with you. Ask them what they want you to know. If you don't get a response right away, don't be discouraged. This is not easy to do at first—it takes practice, time, courage and patience. However, if your sincere intention is to connect and communicate, it will happen. Be patient. If nothing shows up right away, trust when the time is right, when you are completely open to hearing what needs to be communicated, it will be revealed.

There may be times when a word will pop into your head or you simply get a feeling. If you're not sure what's being communicated, rephrase your question into a yes or no format. Until you develop your inner voice, you might also look into some kind of biofeedback system for assistance. Eventually you will discover you have one built in. It's called the parasympathetic nervous system. There are a couple of different ways to measure its response.

One way is to stand with your feet shoulder width apart. Take a couple of breaths and say, "My name is (state your name)." If your body naturally leans forward, that signals a yes. Then make a statement that would naturally produce a no. For instance, you might say, "My name is Donald Duck." Your body should naturally move back, signaling a no.

Another option is muscle testing. Stand with one arm out to your side. Ask a friend to place two fingers on your hand and when a question is asked, apply light pressure. If your arm remains in place, that signifies a yes. If your arm is easily pushed down, that signifies a no. To see if you're doing this exercise properly, again ask if your name is Donald Duck. Your arm should drop to your side when pressure is applied. Believe me, your body knows your name!

There are many books discussing the proper use of these methods. One I recommend highly is Dr. Bradley Nelson's *The Emotion Code*. In addition to the techniques above, Dr. Nelson explains how to move through stuck negative emotions to reach renewed health.

Opening to this type of communication, accepting symptoms as an ally, not an enemy you must destroy, will help immensely in your healing process. Reframe your attitude about your symptoms, look at them as proof your body is working. Form an appreciation for your symptoms and thank them for helping you see where you are out of balance. Above all, be patient and loving with yourself. Learning to listen to your body, learning to trust your intuition takes time. Old habits die hard. But please know, if you are truly interested in healing and changing your life, it is worth the effort.

Being Responsible

When you take responsibility for your life, you are the one in charge. You are the one who gets to decide how to respond to your circumstances. Taking responsibility for your choices requires you to embrace a universal truth that says you participate in the creation of everything in life, including your illness. From this level of awareness, you have the power to choose how to respond.

Owning a part in the creation of your disease does not imply you are guilty of wrongdoing. Please understand that is absolutely not true.

What it says is that by viewing yourself as the center of your universe, the creator of everything in your life, it follows that you also have the power to un-create. I realize this can be a radical thought to many but this model worked for me. I strongly urge you to give this your highest consideration if your intention is to heal.

This concept came to me as an insight during a meditation. Many people who have healed themselves report the same realization and credit this shift in perception as a major step in their healing. Everything that occurs in life exists by divine orchestration. We call forth every situation at the perfect time, according to what is next for us to examine and heal in our life. Nothing is a mistake. There are no accidents and we are not the victim to any circumstance or person. This is evolution of the soul. Sometimes it takes orchestrating a major crisis for us to wake up to our next level of awareness. And though we may see it as a bad thing, the reality is it can be a blessing, a gift in disguise.

Allow Your Body to Do Its Job

When I was first diagnosed, the conventional medical doctors I worked with were very skilled in tracking cancer. That's what they did, and they did it well. They were not concerned with, or trained to look for, the underlying causes of my disease. But cancer is a symptom of a biochemical, emotional, mental and spiritual imbalance. Treating one area can never ensure complete healing. This is the difference between the approach of holistic medicine and that of conventional medicine.

The body's natural motion is in the direction of wellness. That is the design. We are misguided when we think we can regulate our chemical balance with drugs better than through our own innate healing abilities. We are conditioned to attack our symptoms. What I'm talking about is a process of support rather than attack—allowing the body, through its natural ability, to heal the symptoms it is expressing. Throwing drugs at a problem is just adding more poison to an already poisoned system.

The year between losing my left and right breast was proof to me that the approach I was taking was not working. Being told I was healthy and recovering nicely when all along I was getting sicker did not move my healing forward. My doctor was basing his conclusions on the blood tests he was taking every three months. The catch was, he was testing for only a couple of specific things, not to see if my overall biochemical makeup was in balance. Nor was he concerned with my emotional, spiritual, or mental wellbeing. The first thing Dr. Gonzalez did was run a complete hair analysis and blood panel. I was shocked to find how out of balance my physical body was.

I often wonder if in the beginning it was discovered that my biochemical makeup was out of balance and my doctor had started the appropriate treatment, might my experience have been completely different? What if he had suggested I get some counseling to deal with emotional energy patterns that might be blocked and consequently adding to my physical problem? Perhaps if this approach had been used, my body might have had a chance to correct itself. Perhaps I might have been able to avoid losing my breasts. Please be clear, I am not blaming my surgeon. He did his job well. However, if he had been working with a team of doctors that were looking for the underlying physiological problems, things might have been different the second time around.

If you're not in a critical situation with your health, it's a good idea to consult a doctor who can find where your body may be out of balance and get on a program to bring it back. Prevention is healing at its optimum. What I'm talking about is a holistic approach to your health. A practitioner who uses methods of testing to find out where the body is deficient and then uses natural (wherever possible) supplements and herbs to assist the body in regaining balance. The best tests for this are blood panels and hair analysis. And let me reiterate, make sure the lab being used has a good record for accurate testing.

You must also be willing to look at the emotional, mental and spiritual areas of your life. Be conscious that you're not repressing your emotions, that you have a healthy mental attitude and are spiritually connected. You must go beyond your symptoms to the core of what's causing them. Being in touch with your body and intuition is vital to your healing. If you are critically ill, seek out an aggressive holistic physician who has experience with critically ill patients. There is nothing that can substitute for working with someone who has the practical background to meet your specific needs.

Feed Your Body Right

There are more studies coming out all the time that focus on the cumulative effect of eating food that is processed, high in fat, grown in soil that lacks proper nutrients and/or fertilized with pesticides. The results of these studies show these factors can be one of the main causes for serious illnesses that are growing in numbers daily. I am also adding to this list foods that have been genetically modified, since there have been no long-term studies showing the effects of these types of foods and how they might express in the body.

What does this mean? To me it means what goes in my body is extremely important. The good news is I can control that. That's why I do my best everyday to put organic fresh food and purified water into my body.

If you have never tasted organic food, try an organic carrot. Then compare it with one that's been produced with chemical fertilizers. The adulterated carrot tastes bitter, while the organic carrot is sweet and juicy. Get in touch with how your body responds to the difference. As more people demand organic foods, the marketplace will respond by producing more. This will decrease the amount of toxins we ingest on a daily basis.

Look for foods that are "certified organic," meaning they are not grown in chemically treated soil or sprayed with herbicides and pesticides. These toxic chemicals accumulate in our bodies and over time can lead to all manner of health challenges. We must be diligent in the monitoring of our food supply, including GMO foods. We must insist they be labeled so we can make informed choices regarding ingestion of genetically modified foods.

It's a medical fact that it's impossible to maintain a healthy body if you do not feed your cells properly. Eventually the lack of nutrients in the body, along with the cumulative effects of impure food, water, and air will overwhelm your body's ability to handle toxins (poisons) and as a result, your body will begin to break down on a cellular level, making it susceptible to disease. The more junk and toxins we put in our bodies, the more energy our bodies must expend to rid our systems of these foreign invaders. Our poor diets contribute to low energy, depression and a general feeling of subpar health. Something as simple as changing your diet can make a big difference in your energy, vitality and wellbeing.

Changing your diet from inorganic to organic may take a bit of intestinal fortitude (no pun intended), but once your body is released from the need to fight the chemicals and junk coming into it, it is free to work on the backlog of toxins stored there for years.

In other words, you may feel a bit sick at first. Holistic doctors call this a *healing crisis* and consider it good news. It means your body is working. Working in ways it may have never worked before. The symptoms can range from mild flu-like symptoms and nausea to more severe reactions. It depends on how poisoned your body is. Do not be surprised if you get body rashes or pimples where you haven't seen them for years. These symptoms are the result of the body releasing toxins.

During release times, it's good to consult an herbalist who can recommend herbs that support your liver and other elimination organs. Most importantly, try to drink as much purified water as you can. It's a good idea to drink at least two quarts a day of purified water in addition to any other pure organic fruit and vegetable juices.

I personally recommend your fruit or vegetable drinks be juiced at home and not purchased from a store. This is because bottled juices lose a large percentage of their nutrient value within minutes of being processed.

I also recommend you seek a doctor familiar with hair analysis and discuss the results of this test with him/her so you understand what minerals your body might be lacking and what your heavy metal load is. "Heavy metals" is the term used for a group of elements that have particular weight characteristics and are on the "heavier" end of the periodic table of elements. Some heavy metals are essential to our health in trace amounts, while others are nonessential and can even be harmful in excessive amounts. When cancer enters the picture, a body already taxed by heavy metal poisoning can be a ticking time bomb.

Discuss these factors with your doctor in addition to how and why you might need to change your eating habits or add additional supplements and herbs to your diet to bring your body into balance. Pay attention to how your body responds and be sure to monitor your changes with an ongoing series of tests.

Once your test results show you've achieved a greater balance, you will probably be able to back off some of the supplements and/or herbs you are taking. Most importantly, pay attention to how you feel. I can't stress enough how becoming conscious of your life on all levels is key to engaging in a lifestyle that supports a healthier you.

Emotional Balance & Energetic Flow

We understand how toxins enter the body through the food we eat, the air we breathe and the water we drink. But there are other equally threatening toxins that can affect our wellbeing. I'm talking about emotional and mental toxicity that also creates imbalance and ultimately leads to disease.

Because emotions are "energy in motion," when we repress them and stay stuck in negative mental patterns, it creates energy blocks in the body. For many who are familiar with only Western medicine, this is a new concept. But it is not a new science, having been studied by the Chinese for thousands of years.

Our bodies contain biochemical reactions within an electromagnetic field, sometimes referred to as the "body electric." It is that energy that holds not only us together, but the rest of the world as well. Our level of wellness depends on the flow of that energy. Negative emotions or negative mental patterns quite simply stop that flow, creating blocks. Blocked energy weakens the organs associated with the area where energy is stuck, making these organs and areas vulnerable to disease.

There are many ways of alleviating energy blocks. Look for practitioners who work with energy such as Orthogonal chiropractors, network chiropractors, acupuncturists, massage therapists, Reiki masters or Heller workers. Also, remember to check out Dr. Bradley Nelson and his *Emotion Code* method. Doing energy work is yet another facet of your holistic support team but make no mistake—going inward is where real change happens. For me, it was a blessing in disguise that I couldn't afford outside help. It forced me to go inward for my answers.

I have found tremendous solace in prayer. When applied with heartfelt emotion and the trust that what you are asking for is already given, even if it doesn't appear in the form you are expecting, tremendous shifts can happen. It's important to remember the energy you imbue in your prayer helps bring about its manifestation. Prayer is built on belief and faith. Belief is a mental process. Faith is allowing and receiving the desired result into your life as if it has already happened. At the end of your prayer, be sure to thank God for the intervention that is already transpiring.

When praying, be as specific as possible with your request. Detail exactly what you want. I'll never forget the day I asked in prayer for a partner. I listed all the qualities I wanted and then let go, so God could bring him to me. Several months later a man appeared in my life that had every single quality I had asked for. However, he was married. Apparently the only thing I had forgotten to mention was that he be single. So, when praying, be specific!

Another important factor is staying in the present moment. Usually when we're in an emotional state, we are obsessing about something in the past or future. An emotional trigger from our past means we are still carrying baggage around from previous experience. This will affect your physiology. The same is true when we obsess about the future. The present is the only place where power exists, the only place where peace exists.

Being in the moment means focusing on what is right in front of you, in that moment. Make a conscious decision to leave the past behind. Forgive whatever it is in the past that is holding you. Most of us will hold on to negative past experiences over positive ones, because it gives us the illusory feeling of being in control. Consequently, the negative experiences are the ones we obsess over and carry forward in our lives.

Most of these experiences include anger, guilt, shame and vengeance. Usually these negative emotions become convenient weapons to manipulate and control others, particularly those we feel deserve our anger. What we don't consider are the harmful chemical reactions happening in the body when we hold anger and other negative emotions. Adrenaline starts pumping, the heart races and blood pressure rises. This is a natural response set up by the parasympathetic nervous system, commonly known as fight or flight. Used in a momentary crisis, this is an advanced use of the body's self-protective behavior. However, remaining in this state for prolonged periods results in chronic suppression of the immune system, leaving the body vulnerable to dis-ease. Not to mention the incredible amount of energy it takes to remain in this state. Don't get me wrong, all emotions are healthy when expressed properly and released. Get angry, or whatever is appropriate in the moment, express it and move on. It is the persistent inability to let go of negative emotions that creates problems for the body.

When I find myself stuck in negative energy, I often ask in prayer for help in removing it from my body. I close my eyes, imagine what color the emotion is, so I can easily locate it in my body and separate it from the rest of me. Then I imagine a pillar of light in front of me and cast the colored emotion into the light. I then take a moment to replace that energy with love, which for me is the color pink. I fill the void I created with the energy of love and allow it to resonate within my being. Use your imagination and create a technique that works for you. If you're not sure how to get started, ask in prayer or meditation for a symbolic image that will work for you.

The final step to being in the moment is gratitude. Once you release your negative emotions, be thankful for everyone and everything in your life that has gotten you to this point. The more gratitude you express, the more the universe will expand those things for which you are grateful.

I believe everything that happens in our lives happens for a reason. Now, in retrospect, I know all of it is good. I believe if you look back at your life without attachment, you will see everything that has happened to you was perfect and happened for you to grow and evolve. Every experience we have is meant to build character and promote growth. You would not be who you are today without your past. Be grateful for all of it!

If after an honest examination you do not feel this way, I would urge you to reframe your past. Re-imagine how you see things that have happened, rethink your way of viewing ideas, events, situations or experiences you've had. Review your perceptions and see if there's another way to hold your thoughts around whatever you're trying to heal. Reframing allows you to view yourself as strong and courageous for having survived your trials as opposed to feeling victimized by them. It is a method of using the whole truth and not just our limited understanding of it.

Clarity

A wonderful side effect of all the work I did on myself was the resultant clarity I experienced. One of the things I realized when I began to expel the toxic substances from my body, including my toxic emotions and beliefs, was that I felt clear for the first time in my life. My senses were heightened beyond anything I had experienced before.

Before embarking on this journey, I was always confused about what to do or where to go. Simple decisions were difficult for me. I didn't have a clear view of what was in front of me, or what to do about it. I think a lot of people go through life with dulled senses and fuzzy thinking, constantly questioning their decisions. There may be other causes such as low self-esteem or insecurity, but a wonderful side effect of achieving clarity is that it automatically creates confidence and a higher sense of wellbeing.

As with everything, the process of pursuing clarity induces change. You might find yourself needing to give up toxic relationships, move out of toxic environments or unable to eat most fast foods! In other words, your whole life is going to change. But that is the good news that comes with a ticket to a healthier you!

Resistance/Surrender

I'd like to wrap up with one of the most difficult pills to swallow. Change. It's an interesting phenomenon that even when faced with a life-threatening situation, we are still resistant to change. Even when we understand it intellectually, our struggle with it is so embedded in our psyches that we cannot identify it as the major pitfall it is to achieving and maintaining our health and peace of mind.

Change brings up fear. Even when the habits and patterns of our lives are destructive, we tend to stay stuck in those patterns. We like it because it's familiar. We would rather stay in a toxic relationship because we're afraid we can't make it on our own. We fear what will become of us so we choose to stay with the devil we know rather than risk the devil we don't know, assuming that change will surely bring an even more robust devil.

Pay attention to what you resist. Use your resistance as a tool to identify the areas in your life that need examination. Change, as difficult as it seems, is what life is all about. In fact, the only constant is change. To resist it is to create a life filled with pain and struggle.

When you find yourself resisting change, unable to cope with the resultant disastrous outcomes, it should serve as a red flag to pay attention. By resisting change or remaining stuck in your dis-ease, you guarantee the lessons around your issues will come back again and again, probably at a much higher cost. One thing I learned from three bouts of cancer is that *when the Universe wants our attention, it will continue sending the same message in ever-increasing intensity until we get it.*

The mind is great at convincing us to play it safe, using fear and resistance as its messengers. One way to deal with resistance is to ask, "What am I afraid of?" Once you've identified your fear, ask,

"Is this fear real?" It has been my experience that nine times out of ten, the answer is an unqualified, "No!" Fear is an illusion based on an unknowable future. A future we cannot possibly predict. It follows then that if it is not real, there is nothing to fear, or resist.

Surrender your resistance to the Divine Spirit, that unlimited part of you that knows all. Make a commitment to "Let go and Let God." Acknowledge that control is an illusion and resistance is futile. Only in this truth will you find freedom from worry and make way for the perfect unfolding of your life.

If you're ready to stop struggling, to embrace a healthier way of being, I invite you to release your need to control the direction of your life. Surrender to a higher power. It is the only force that truly knows what you need to evolve into your highest and best.

Life is a gift, regardless of its packaging. Embrace this truth. It will bring you peace. And in this peace, you will find healing. *Namaste*.

About the Authors

Brenda Michaels

Brenda Michaels is currently the co-host of *Conscious Talk . . . Radio that Makes a Difference*, with her husband and partner in all things, Rob Spears. In her role as National Speaker, Workshop Leader and one-on-one coach to cancer patients, she is grateful to share the insights gained from her own healing experience while reminding herself and others that life is a work in progress. Brenda is a fierce advocate for animal rights and a student of her two amazing cats, who have taught her that "playtime" is as important to her as it is to them. They all harmoniously share a home in Washington State. You can visit her website at *www.intentionalshift.com*

Marsha Mercant

Marsha Mercant is a multi-award-winning actor/singer and voice-over artist who has performed internationally on stage as well as in film and television. Turning her creative passion to writing, Marsha was co-editor and contributor to the Amazon #1 Bestseller *Fearless Women, Visions of a New World*. With the formation of *Write To Speak LLC*, Marsha expanded her writing to include the editing and co-writing of several books, both fiction and nonfiction. With the completion of her new play, *When You Get There*, she adds playwright to her many accomplishments. Marsha lives with her dashing husband and perfect dog in New Jersey. You can visit her website at *www.writetospeak.com*